How to Have a

HEALTHY
PREGNANCY,
HEALTHY
BIRTH

With
Traditional Chinese Medicine

REVISED EDITION

by

Honora Lee Wolfe

BLUE POPPY PRESS

Published by:

Blue Poppy Press
1775 Linden Ave.
Boulder, CO 80304
(303) 447-8372

First Edition January, 1993
Second Printing June, 1994

ISBN 0-936185-40-6
Library of Congress #-92-75778

COMP Designation: Original work

Printed on recycled paper at Westview Press, Boulder, CO. ✪
Cover printed at C & M Press, Thornton, CO.

10, 9, 8, 7, 6, 5, 4, 3

Preface

P regnancy — so much has been said and written about this seemingly inexhaustible topic. Both men and women are endlessly fascinated with the process by which new life develops and is brought into the world. As much as we know about the biology of it, the miracle of it is always unfathomable. It is a wonderful, everyday miracle, and one in which a woman gets to be a central participant. Thus, for most women, pregnancy is a blessed event, greatly to be desired. Despite discomforts which can and, often do, accompany this part of a woman's life cycle, most women find pregnancy to be exciting, an adventure to be embraced, a time of joy and anticipation. It is the purpose of this book to enhance this adventure of pregnancy and birth through the wisdom of Chinese medicine.

Historically, the hallmark of Chinese medicine is the emphasis it places on prevention as opposed to merely remedial care. The *Nei Jing*, the earliest classic of Chinese medicine, states that treating disease after it has arisen is the lowest level of health care and treatment. Consequently, traditional Chinese doctors have spent considerable time and energy discovering and elucidating the laws governing the maintenance of health from every point of view: climate, diet, lifestyle, psychology, sociology, sex, and hygiene.

Central to the Oriental notion of natural law is the idea that the beginning of any event greatly determines the subsequent development and outcome of that event. Therefore the conception, gestation, birth, and postpartum care of an individual have vast implications for that person's subsequent health, happiness, and social adjustment. Chinese doctors have developed a system of pre and postnatal care based on their interpretation of natural law which is preventive, low cost, humane, ethical, and most of all, effective.

This book is an introduction to these Chinese teachings concerning pregnancy, birth, and postpartum care written for the general reader. As such, it is a companion volume to two other Blue Poppy Press editions written for professional practitioners of Traditional Chinese Medicine (TCM), *Path of Pregnancy, Vol. I: A Handbook of Traditional Chinese Gestational & Birthing Diseases*, and *Path of Pregnancy, Vol. II: A Handbook of Traditional Chinese Postpartum Diseases*. This updated edition has some new information not in the first edition, written in late 1992. We have also corrected minor errors and clarified some points which we felt were not explained as well as they might be. It is my hope that this information may provide new insights and options for all prospective parents and parents-to-be, as well as healthy and happy babies.

Honora Lee Wolfe
June 16, 1994

Contents

Introduction

T hroughout Chinese history, successful pregnancy and birth have been of the utmost importance. Healthy heirs ensured the continuity of the family, the honoring of the ancestors, and the future of the empire. Also, as in most agrarian cultures, abundant children provided a ready workforce as well as a social security system. Finally, as mentioned in the preface, the beginning of life was believed to be of great portent concerning the development and success of a person's entire life. Therefore, much has been written on these subjects in Chinese medical texts over the centuries.

Some Chinese medical ideas that you will encounter in this book may sound archaic or peculiar. However, it must be noted that there are more Chinese people on the planet than any other single race or nationality. This fact alone lends credibility to their medical practices. Furthermore, Chinese medical practices related to pregnancy and birth have been used for over two millennia. Knowing the Chinese to be very practical people, we can assume that they would not continue to use a system of health care that was not effective. Therefore, in reading this book, I would ask the reader to keep an open mind concerning ideas or practices that sound foreign or old-fashioned.

Chinese medicine is based upon a very different conceptual paradigm than modern biomolecular medicine. This fact does not render it less valid or true. Consider an analogy using maps. Although mapping the same territory, a rainfall map looks very different from a road map or a topographical map. However, the information on one map does not invalidate the information on the other. They are merely mapping the same territory in different ways. So it is with Chinese medicine and modern Western medicine. Each is true according to its own set of parameters, and must be viewed and judged by those parameters alone. It is best not to try to cross reference one to the other. For you, the reader, to view the Chinese medical "map" effectively, there are several key terms and ideas used throughout the book that must first be introduced.

Chinese Medical Ideas Related to Pregnancy

Some readers may be familiar with the ideas presented in this section. For others, these words and ideas may be new and foreign. If you have difficulty understanding at first, it may be useful to reread parts of this section as the words or ideas are brought up in later chapters.

Yin & Yang

Yin and yang are terms in Chinese philosophy and medicine used to describe the polarization of all phenomena in the universe. As such, a basic understanding of yin and yang is vital to understanding Chinese medicine. As a result of the constant flux and interplay of these two opposing/complementary forces, all things evolve and devolve, arise and disappear.

In the West, these words have been used in many erroneous ways, and there are many misconceptions as to their meaning. I will try to present these important concepts as clearly as possible in relationship to Chinese medicine as a whole.

First, yin and yang are generic terms describing opposing aspects or phenomena in nature. They may be used to represent any two opposing objects or ideas, or opposite aspects within a single object or idea.

In all situations, yin and yang are interdependent. One does not, indeed cannot, exist without the other, just as dark implies light. Through opposition they create unity.

The relationship of yin and yang is in constant flux within a living being or system, just as the seasons follow each other. Although health is relative balance of yin and yang, this is never a static balance.

In the human body or in nature, two natural symbols guide the classification of all other phenomena into yin and yang categories. These are fire and water. Fire represents yang; water represents yin. Any object that has properties or causes energetic change similar to those of fire and water is described similarly as predominantly yang or yin.

Yin and yang are only relative concepts. An object or phenomenon can be yin in one situation or comparison, and yang in another. They are not absolute, nor do they imply any value judgement.

Within the body it is said that qi (movement and function) is yang in relationship to blood (substance and nourishment) and that *jing* (primal substance) is yin in relationship to spirit (primal movement). Within the body yin and yang must remain in dynamic, harmonious balance. Yang must quicken yin; yin must nourish, cool, and root yang. Life requires them both, as the seed sprouts in spring only with the nourishment of the soil and melting snow (yin) and the warmth of the sun (yang).

If the harmonious relationship of interpromotion and restraint is lost in the body or in nature, disorder and discomfort arise. The chart below shows some pairs of basic yin/yang polarities. However, in looking at this chart, it is important to remember that these yin/yang dichotomies only describe the relationship between the two opposites given. Darkness is yin only in comparison with light. It in no way implies that females are dark and males are light or that females are calm and males are agitated. Nothing is inherently yin or yang; something is more yin or more yang only in relationship to something else. Ultimately, there is no thing that is yin or yang. Yin/yang theory is only a mental conceptualization created by the ancient Chinese to organize their description of reality. It is no different from the mathematics of 0 and 1 used to program computers.

Yang	Yin
Fire	**Water**
Heaven	Earth
Day	Night
Spring/Summer	Autumn/Winter
Male	Female
Hot	Cold
Light	Darkness
Light	Heavy
Upward/Outward	Downward/Inward
Surface	Bones
Bowels	Organs
Function	Form or Substance
Movement	Stillness

Qi, Blood, & *Jing*

While these Chinese terms are difficult to translate, we can get an idea of their meaning by considering their functions in the body.

Qi

In most English language books on Chinese medicine, writers and translators render the word qi as energy, but this is not quite correct. A more exact translation, which has been used by a few translators, is the word influences[1]. Another doctor has tried to make the idea of qi clear by describing it this way:

> The concept of qi is unlimited. Any movement, no matter how small or how large, how brief or how long, how quick or how slow is caused by qi. When qi concentrates it is called matter, and where it spreads it is called space. When qi gathers together it is called life, and when it separates it is called death. When qi flows it is called health and when it is blocked there is disease.
>
> Planets depend upon it for their brightness. Weather is formed by it. The seasons are caused by it. Man cannot stand outside of qi. It supports him and permeates him as water is contained within the ocean.[2]

While this poetic description gives one some idea of the difficulty in translating Chinese medical terminology, the easiest way to under-

---

[1] Unschuld, Paul U., *Medicine in China, A History of Ideas*, University of California Press, Berkeley, 1985, p. 67-68

[2] Dr. Liang, as quoted in a correspondance course from the North American Academy of Acupuncture and Moxibustion, Portland, OR, from the mid 1970's, no longer in existance.

stand the concept of qi is that qi is function (as opposed to structure). It is yang in relationship to blood being yin. In the body, all physiological activity is described by and dependent upon the movements and mutations of qi. The five intrinsic characteristics of qi are:

1. Movement or propulsion: Qi propels the blood, transports nutritive substance to the entire body, and circulates body fluid.

2. Warming: Qi maintains the body temperature and by its warming nature energizes all the functional activities of the organism.

3. Defense: Qi defends the body surface against invasion by external pathogens.

4. Transformation: Qi transforms the blood and body fluids. It creates these from the raw materials derived from respiration and digestion.

5. Restraint or astringency: The Qi holds the blood within its vessels, the body fluids within the body, and the organs up against gravity.

Blood

Described as the substance that flows through the vessels, its main function is to nourish all parts of the body. It is more substantial than qi. In the *Nei Jing,* it says that "The qi commands the blood; the blood is the mother of the qi." This statement describes the basic relationship of qi and blood and the yin/yang polarity between them. While the qi is responsible for the movement, warmth, transformation, and restraint of the blood, blood is the underlying nourishment that allows the qi these functions. Without blood or nourishment (yin), the qi (yang) is without root, substantial foundation, or mother. Without qi (yang) to move, warm, and transform it, the blood (yin) is inert, without force or direction. The blood is the nutritive substance that the qi then consumes, transforms, or evaporates to create function. As always, yin and yang are completely interdependent and interpromoting.

Jing

Jing refers to the vital physical essence of the body, its seminal basis. It is the primary substantial element responsible for determining physical growth, development, and maintenance of life activity and metabolism. The outward physical manifestation of *jing* in women is menstrual blood: in men it is semen. It is the material base necessary for the creation of a new being, the creation of life. Therefore, *jing* essence is yin in relationship to spirit, which is the non-material or yang impetus necessary for the creation of life.

These three terms, qi, blood, and *jing*, will come up repeatedly in this book, since they are the stuff from which life is created.

Conception

In the days when traditional Chinese medical theory was first written down, doctors did not have microscopes or laboratory tests. Chinese doctors could not see sperm or eggs. Their description of conception, based solely upon what they knew or could see with the naked eye, is different from Western medicine's. They could see that both babies and menstrual blood came out of the womb. They knew that women cannot become pregnant before menarche or after the menopause. They could see the male ejaculate and knew that men must ejaculate into the woman for her to become pregnant. They therefore assumed that the ejaculate in the man and the blood in the female respectively were the reproductive essences (*jing*). These sexual or reproductive essences of the parents that combine to form the fertilized zygote are poetically described as "the red and the white essences."

Chinese medicine says that healthy essence, male and female, makes healthy babies. Good red essence, or blood, should be like liquid paint or hare's blood, not dark, heavy, or clotted. Good white essence, or semen, should be white, heavy, sweet, and abundant. For 2,000 years or more, prospective parents in China have taken Chinese medicine to insure that their reproductive essence is strong and that, therefore, their children will also be strong and healthy. Such treatment is still available and is a large part of the Chinese medical treatment of both male and female infertility.

After conception, the united red and white essence congeal to become the embryo in the womb.[3] Chinese medicine has a great deal to say about the womb or uterus.

The Uterus

In Chinese medicine the uterus has many names. The most common name is the *bao gong* or wrapper palace. The uterus is a very special organ in Chinese medicine. It is one of the so-called eight extraordinary bowels. To understand the eight extraordinary bowels, one must first have some idea about the organs and bowels according to Chinese medicine. This is because their definitions and functions are very different from those of modern Western medicine. Again, we encounter a different map.

In Chinese medicine, there are five solid organs (liver, heart, spleen, lungs, kidneys) and 6 hollow bowels (gall bladder, small intestine, stomach, large intestine, urinary bladder, triple heater). The primary function of the solid organs is to create, receive, and store pure

---

[3]   Chang Huang, *Du Shu Pian*, trans. by Paul V. Unschuld, excerpted in *Introductory Readings in Classical Chinese Medicine*, Kluwer Academic Publishers, Dordrecht, Boston, London, 1988, p. 57

substances (blood, liquids, qi, *jing* or essence). They store and do not discharge. The primary function of the hollow bowels is to transport and discharge both pure substances and waste materials. The uterus is an extraordinary bowel because in form it is hollow, like a bowel. Also like a bowel, it discharges the menstruate and, at the appropriate time, the fully developed fetus. However, it also functions like a solid organ, receiving the female reproductive essence (*jing*) and storing the fetus for 10 lunar months.

Not only does the uterus store and then discharge the fetus and the menstruate, it also functions as part of the body's communication network, which we will discuss later.

Gestation

At the moment of fertilization, the zygote is endowed with what is called *yuan qi*, usually translated as source qi. Source qi can be seen as one's constitutional vigor or genetic inheritance. Original qi is finite in amount and kind and cannot be altered or augmented. It is the catalyst for all metabolic activity throughout life and is responsible for the initial growth and development of the embryo until the placenta is formed.

As the embryo grows and the placenta develops, there is a tremendous increase in blood production in the mother's body. This increase in blood production is required to nourish the growing child.

There are several organs and channels in the body that participate in the production and circulation of this blood. According to Chinese medicine, blood is manufactured by the spleen from the purest part of the food and liquids that we ingest. This pure substance is sent to the heart where, according to the classical literature, it is turned red. It is the heart's job to then send the blood down to the uterus, via a very important internal channel called the *chong mai*, or sometimes the *bao mai*. Often called the penetrating vessel or the sea of blood, this channel is very important during pregnancy and to all female reproductive functions. It is thought of as running up and down the central core of the body. The other important channel in the body during gestation is the *ren mai*, or conception vessel, which runs up and down the ventral or front surface of the body from the mouth to the vagina. It is often said that the qi in the *ren mai* controls the blood in the *chong mai*. Again we have a yin/yang polarity.

It is via the *chong mai* that the heart and uterus communicate, and qi and blood can and does flow in either direction through it at different times in a woman's reproductive life cycle. This becomes even more interesting when considering the emotions of the mother during pregnancy. In Chinese medicine each organ is said to house or have a relationship to a certain aspect of the psyche. It is the heart that houses the *shen* or spirit. It is important for spirit to rest calmly in the heart in order for the heart to perform its duties properly. That is one reason there is such an emphasis in Chinese medicine for mothers to be calm, rested, and not to be frightened. Fright, anxiety, or fatigue might injure the heart spirit and compromise the communication between the heart and uterus, which is so important to the development of the child.

In addition to the blood created by the spleen and sent to the uterus by the heart via the *bao mai*, the embryo or fetus requires substantial amounts of the mother's *jing* or vital essence during its development. The kidneys are responsible for storing the body's *jing*. It is transported to the uterus via another internal channel called the *bao luo*, or wrapper connecting vessel. According to Wang Yao-ting, the *bao*

10

luo refers to the passages distributed over the *bao gong* (uterus) which fill it with life essence from the kidneys.[4]

Above, I mentioned that the uterus also plays a role in the communication of the organs in the body. All the organs and bowels must be in communication with each other for the body to remain healthy. The link between the heart and kidneys is especially vital. That is because the heart is the main representative of fire (yang), and the kidneys are the main representative of water (yin) in the body. Water and fire must mutually control each other if the body is to remain healthy. If they come out of balance, many types of problems may arise. However, there is a specific pattern of disharmony in Chinese medicine called *heart and kidneys not communicating*. Since the heart and kidney communicate through the uterus via the network of the *bao luo* and *bao mai*, this function of the uterus is very important for the life-long health of a woman. It is, therefore, very important for women to avoid unnecessary hysterectomies. Happily, Chinese medicine has effective treatments for many conditions for which hysterectomies are the Western medical treatment of choice.

Returning to the developing fetus, we have said that the fetus is nourished by blood created by the spleen and sent to the uterus by the heart and that it is maintained by the life essence (*jing*) from the kidneys. However, the spleen and kidneys each have yet another job to do in relationship to the growing fetus. In the section on qi, we described one of the qi's jobs as restraint. Here restraint means holding up the organs against gravity. In relation to the fetus growing in the uterus, it is the spleen qi that must do this job. If a woman has problems of the fetus falling out of the uterus, it is the spleen qi that

---

4   Wang Yao-ting, "A Preliminary Discussion of the *Bao Gong, Bao Mai, & Bao Luo*, trans. by Zhang Ting-liang & Bob Flaws, appearing in *Blue Poppy Essays, 1988*, Blue Poppy Press, Boulder, CO, 1988, p. 18-19

must be boosted to prevent this. Thus, we can see that a strong spleen is quite important for a healthy pregnancy.

It is the kidneys, on the other hand, which are responsible for a function that, in Chinese, is called *gu*. This word means to consolidate. During pregnancy, besides providing *jing* to the growing child, the kidneys must *gu* the fetus. That is, they must consolidate or contain the fetus firmly in the uterus.

So far we have considered the uterus, heart, spleen, kidneys, and internal channels in relationship to pregnancy. However, there is one more organ that requires at least a brief mention before we go on, and that is the liver. The liver has two important jobs that are vital to a successful pregnancy and birth.

First, it is said that the liver stores the blood. This does not necessarily mean that blood is stored *in* the liver, only *by* the liver. The *chong mai* is sometimes called the sea of blood and the uterus as the blood chamber, but it is the liver that stores the blood there. Since it is blood that nourishes the fetus, the liver's role here is quite important.

The second job of the liver is that is it is in charge of coursing and discharge. This means that the liver governs the smooth and free flow of qi through the body. Since it is the qi that moves the blood, if the qi flows freely, the blood is more likely to do so as well. If the liver qi is not free flowing for some reason, then the blood in the body is less likely to be free flowing. This free flowing quality is important to insure a healthy, continuous supply of blood to the uterus and *chong mai*. Also, free flowing liver qi is important when it comes time for the child to be born. Tight, congested liver qi can make labor more painful and lengthen its duration. Thus, we see the importance of a relaxed and healthy liver. This is discussed again later in the chapters on prevention and self care, and the chapter on postpartum problems.

Stasis & Stagnation

The Chinese medical idea of stagnation and stasis is a very important factor in problems during pregnancy. Stagnation describes any qi or substance in the body that is not flowing properly and therefore getting stuck. Six things can become stagnant in the body according to Chinese medicine: qi, blood, food, dampness, phlegm, and fire, and a stagnation of one of these can lead to or exacerbate stagnation of any of the others. During pregnancy, the growing fetus is pressing on the abdominal organs and diminishing the available spaces through which qi, blood, and body fluids may flow. Therefore, even the healthiest of women is more susceptible to stagnation during gestation.

Stagnation and stasis contribute to many problems both during and after pregnancy, and again this will be discussed more in later chapters.

The above are the basic terms and concepts necessary to understand conception, pregnancy, and birth, as well as problems that may arise during these processes according to Chinese medicine. Since these ideas are referred to throughout this book, the reader should refer to this chapter as necessary. At the least, the reader should see that the world of Chinese medicine has little to do with the world of modern Western medicine. However, just as two different maps of a single terrain are valid from their own points of view, Chinese medicine is as valid and true as is modern Western medicine. It is merely a different map or paradigm of the body and its functions. Chinese medicine has been proven effective by well over 100 generations of Chinese physicians.

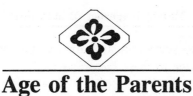

Age of the Parents

T here are many factors to consider when deciding the best time to have a child or how to space them if one intends to have two or more. Assuming that a child is not a fortuitous accident and that a couple has a choice in deciding when is the best time physically, social and financial factors will also play a part in such decisions. While younger parents have more physical vigor and stamina, older parents may be more mature, stable, and financially secure.

The Chinese classics say that ideally the father should be 30 years old and the mother 20. Of course these ages are based upon a traditional culture with clearly defined sexual roles. While this is hardly the case in late 20th century America, let us consider these ages from a more traditional point of view.

By 30 years a man should be at his physical peak, established in his career, and a stable, responsible provider, if indeed he ever will be. At 20, the woman is full of abundant qi, blood, and *jing*. As we have seen from the discussions in the previous chapter, the developing fetus requires these three substances in large amounts. The older the woman, the more likely it is that she will have problems due to blood and yin vacuity during and after the pregnancy. These may include difficulty conceiving, possible miscarriage, and various postpartum difficulties.

While there is probably little difference between the energetic health of a woman 20 or 25, this difference is considerable by the time a woman reaches her mid 30's. By that time, a woman's production of blood and yin has begun to decline. Additionally, since people are more susceptible to stasis and stagnation as they age, problems may arise more easily due to these factors as well.

By a woman's early 40's, pregnancy and birth become even more difficult and even hazardous for both mother and child. It is interesting that the incidence of Down's syndrome and other birth defects rises steeply for children of mothers over 40. According to Chinese medicine, most such defects are due to an insufficiency of inherited *jing* from the parents.

Keeping all this in mind, Chinese medicine suggests that the older the mother, the more preventive care before, during, and after the pregnancy she will require.

Clearly, decisions about when to have children involve many complex factors, not just the age of the parents. In fact, many women may not have the luxury to decide at what age to conceive. Whatever age a woman is when she becomes pregnant, however, Chinese medicine has a great deal to offer her in the way of both preventive and remedial care. This insures the health of both the mother and child.

In terms of spacing of pregnancies, the considerations are quite similar: how quickly a woman can recuperate her blood and *jing* to be as healthy as possible for another pregnancy. This is based upon her age, constitution, and general health. Some Chinese doctors believe that 5 years between pregnancies allows the woman to recuperate her yin energies fully. However, this basically means raising each child separately. Children close in age play with each other, keep each other occupied, and are therefore less demanding than the solitary child who relates primarily to his or her parents. On the other hand, an older child, say seven to ten years older, can be a significant help in raising a younger sibling. There are no guidelines here. However, if a woman knows the health factors involved, she and her family can make more educated decisions that are sensible for their situation. Since younger women recuperate more quickly and easily than older women, it can be said that young women can have babies in quicker succession with fewer problems and faster recuperation than older women.

The Timing of Conception

I f a couple knows that they wish to become pregnant, there are several specific times during which, according to Chinese medicine, conception may prove unhealthy for the child and are, therefore, to be avoided. They are:

- at noon
- at midnight
- during a solar eclipse
- during a thunder and lightning storm
- during a lunar eclipse
- during a rainbow
- at the summer or winter solstice
- at the full moon
- when either intoxicated or with a full stomach[1]
- during a woman's menstruation
- while either partner is suffering from a skin disease
- while in mourning
- during or for 100 days after having a hot or warm disease
- while distressed or in shock

---

[1]   Lu, Dr. Henry C., *Chinese Secrets of Human Sexuality,* course materials, Lesson 10, p. 17. The consequences, according to the Yellow Emperor, take place at these times and are: 1)noon - child will vomit a lot; 2)midnight - child will be deaf and/or a mute; 3)solar eclipse - child will be weak; 4)lightning and thunder - child will be insane; 5)lunar eclipse -both mother and child will experience bad luck; 7)winter or summer solstice - mother and child will both suffer; 8)full moon - child will be plagued by eye diseases; 9)intoxicated or with indigestion - child will have a tendency to insanity, carbuncles, or piles

The first eight of these are times when yin and yang are in great flux and the climatic or macrocosmic energies are highly polarized. Since the energy of the human body is a microcosm of the larger external macrocosm, such times of disequilibrium could lead to an inherent energetic imbalance in the constitution of a child conceived at such a time. This is based on the idea that any two events that happen simultaneously share the same qi or *zeitgeist*. The Chinese idea of health is based upon moderation and the doctrine of the mean, as is all Chinese culture. Any extreme is seen as fraught with peril. A child conceived at such a time would tend to be special, peculiar, out of the ordinary and interesting. They could be exceedingly good or bad depending upon the circumstances. It is just that special people have special problems.

The injunction against conception while one of the two partners is suffering from a skin disease is quite interesting. From the Chinese medical point of view, many skin diseases are the result of heat in the blood. This heat may be passed to the child with the parent's *jing* where it is latent or hidden. This latent or hidden heat is called *tai du*, translated as fetal toxins, and can cause several childhood diseases that we will discuss in a later section.

The proscription against conception during and for 100 days after a warm or hot disease is similar in reasoning to that of skin diseases, described above. Warm diseases, or *wen bing*, can cause fetal toxins by endowing the fertilized zygote with latent heat that will cause disease processes during early childhood. Another way to think about this is that warm diseases are yang in nature. A yang disease process often may harm the yin of the body, including the blood and *jing*. Since these yin substances are the substrates or foundations for conception, any disease process that harms them should be fully resolved before conception.

20

The best time for conception to take place is after midnight, around the time of the first cock crow.[2] This would be between 3-5 AM, or just before dawn. A child conceived at this time is believed to be intelligent, energetic, relaxed, and beautiful. This is because the macrocosmic energy at this time of day is very balanced yin to yang, but the yang is in ascendency or beginning to grow. Since growth and development are inherently yang in nature, this time is considered auspicious for the conception of a new life that now must grow and develop in the mother's womb.

---

[2]   Ibid., p. 17

Determining Gender

I n traditional Chinese society, the sex of the child was very important for the family. Because of this, astrologers and physicians in ancient times spent a good deal of energy creating charts and mathematical systems to allow a family to find out the sex of the child already conceived, or to try to conceive a child at a certain time to insure the birth of either a boy or girl. These calculations involved yin or yang aspects of the lunar month and year, and the age of the mother at the time of conception.

Additionally, it is thought that specific sexual techniques could increase one's odds of establishing a specific gender of the child. Since the male sperm are more yang, it is quicker and more lively, but not as long-lived as the female sperm that are yin. The yin sperm are slower, but tend to survive longer. Therefore, ejaculation with shallow insertion is more likely to result in a male if intercourse takes place after ovulation since the male sperm can cover a short distance faster than the female sperm. Deep insertion after ovulation will place a higher percentage of slower female sperm in the vicinity of the egg. This gives the female sperm a better chance. Before ovulation, the situation is reversed since the female sperm will have a better chance to survive and make contact with the egg as it descends.

While the ancient Chinese ideas on this topic are quite interesting, it is unlikely that more than a handful of readers will find this information useful or practicable. Furthermore, there is no way to be assured of the accuracy of this material. It may be interesting, however, to note that some Chinese doctors feel that they can tell the sex of the child based upon reading the mother's pulse at the radial artery on the wrist.

In general, most women's pulses get larger and stronger with pregnancy and are not as deep as usual. It is believed that if the overall pulse on the left wrist is larger, this denotes a boy. A larger overall pulse on the right foretells a girl. Further, if the pulse is larger in the distal or inch position (closest to the hand), this suggests a boy; whereas, a larger proximal or foot position (closer to the elbow) indicates a girl.

Classical Theory on Development
of the Fetus in Utero

A ccording to classical Chinese medical theory, certain types of fetal development take place during certain months of gestation. Concomitantly, it was believed that certain activities should be encouraged or avoided by the mother and that certain types of therapy were either useful or to be avoided. While some of these ideas may sound old-fashioned, it seems to me useful to present the material, at least briefly, for historical purposes alone. Furthermore, some of this material may ring true for some women or provide some insight that improves the quality of pregnancy for them. The material here is translated and paraphrased from the *Qian Jin Yao Fang*, by Sun Si-miao, a famous doctor of the Tang Dynasty period, 618-907 CE (AD). When Dr. Sun speaks of months, he is referring to lunar months. Words in parentheses have been added by the author.

The first month of pregnancy is called embryonic beginnings. (There will be a) preference for delicacies and foods that are sour and delicious. While it is appropriate to eat wheat, no strong-smelling acrid foods are to be consumed. This is (the time of) rectifying poor habits. (The mother) should not engage in vigorous activity, sleep should be restful and quiet, and fear should be avoided. An excess of cold will cause pain, while an excess of heat will cause sudden fright, severe abdominal pain, abdominal fullness, and urinary urgency.

The second month of pregnancy is referred to as beginning to gel. Spicy and rancid foods should be avoided. One should live in a quiet residence and be undisturbed by males.[1] It is during the second month that the child's essence takes shape inside the uterine lining. Care should be taken to protect against fright. During the second month of pregnancy, yin and yang begin to occupy the channels and if there is an excess of cold, there will be a miscarriage. If there is heat, (the fetus will) wither.

The third month of pregnancy is referred to as fetal beginnings. During this time, no formalities should be observed and one should adapt to situations as they present themselves. If one wants a male child, hold a bow and arrow, while if one wants a female child, then handle pearls.[2] If one wants a beautiful and good child, then repeatedly touch a jade seal. If one desires a virtuous and good child then one should sit formally with a clear and empty mind. This is called "external symbols having internal influences." During this month, the heart channel is being nourished, and so acupuncture/moxibustion should not be performed on this channel.

During the fourth month of pregnancy, the fetus receives the water essence and blood vessels develop. Rice and fish broth should be eaten. This is referred to as "the development of blood and qi, penetrating to the ears and eyes, and circulating throughout the channels and connecting vessels." It is during the fourth month that the child's six organs normally develop. One should calm one's body, harmonize one's mind and ambition, and regulate one's diet.

During the fifth month of pregnancy, the fetus receives the fire essence and this becomes qi. Arise early and bathe. Wear clear

---

[1]   The implication here is that sexual intercourse should be avoided.

[2]   It is interesting to note here that it was believed that the sex of the child could still be changed or manipulated as late as this in the pregnancy.

clothing and have a clean residence and wear a substantial amount of clothing as well. In the morning inhale the heavenly brightness (*i.e.*, sun oneself) and avoid contraction of colds. Eat rice and wheat, turnips, beef, and mutton. This is called nourishing the qi so as to fix the five organs. During the fifth month of pregnancy the foot *tai yin* vessel is being nourished and acupuncture/moxibustion may not be performed on this channel. Foot *tai yin* is connected internally with the spleen, and it is during the fifth month that the infant's extremities develop. Therefore, (the mother) should not become excessively hungry or overeat. She should avoid consumption of dry foods, not be exposed to baking heat, and not become excessively fatigued.

During the sixth month of pregnancy, the metal essence begins to be received and this develops the sinews.[3] The body should have some slight exertion (and) a quiet house is not so necessary. She should eat muscular fowl and the flesh of fierce beasts. She should be out in the fields watching running animals and horses. During the sixth month of pregnancy, the foot *yang ming* channel is being nourished and acupuncture/moxibustion may not be performed on this channel. Foot *yang ming* is associated internally with the stomach and oversees the mouth and eyes. It is during the sixth month that the mouth and eyes develop, so the five tastes should be regulated, food should be sweet and delicious, and one should not overeat.

During the seventh month of pregnancy, the fetus receives the water essence, which is what becomes the bones. (The mother should) continue to moderately exert herself and move her limbs, since stretching movements circulate the qi and blood. Certainly at this time, one should live in a dry residence and avoid cold food and drink, typically eating rice and keeping one's pores closed. This is referred to as "nourishing the bone and hardening the teeth." It is

---

[3]   Connective tissue

during the seventh month that the child's skin and hair develop. Do not yell a great deal or cry out; do not wear light clothes, and do not bathe or drink cold fluids.

During the eighth month of pregnancy, the fetus receives the earth essence and this forms the skin (literally the hide or leather). The mind should be peaceful and rested, not causing extremes in the movement of qi. This is referred to as "compacting the striae of the skin to make them lustrous." During the eighth month of pregnancy, the hand *yang ming* is being nourished and acupuncture/moxibustion may not be performed on this channel. Hand *yang ming* is internally related to the large intestine that governs the nine orifices. It is during this time that the nine orifices are formed. One should not eat dry foods and not inadvertently miss meals.

During the ninth month of pregnancy, the fetus receives the stone essence which becomes the skin and the hair, the six viscera and the myriad articulations, and all (development) is completed. One should drink sweet wine, eat sweet food, and keep one's belt loose. This is called nourishing the hair (and) augmenting intelligence. During the ninth month of pregnancy, the foot *shao yin* vessel is nourished and so there can be no acupuncture/moxibustion performed on this channel. Foot *shao yin* is connected internally to the kidneys and the kidneys control the continuity (of the generations). It is during the ninth month that all the child's vessels become continuous. Do not dwell in (excessively) warm or chilled places or touch baked clothing.

During the tenth month of pregnancy, the five organs are complete, the six bowels are connected. The qi of heaven and earth has been absorbed into the cinnabar field.[4] Therefore, everything is unified and the personal spirit is complete and only delivery remains.

The above material gives the reader a glimpse of some classical Chinese ideas about pregnancy, proper behavior and diet for the mother, and the concept of fetal education, which is the subject of an entire chapter below.

[4]   This term refers to the lower abdomen which is seen as the root of the body.

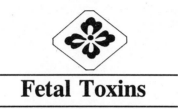

Fetal Toxins

A s mentioned above in the section on the timing of conception, there is a theory in Chinese medicine about the source of many early childhood illnesses which has no analog in Western medicine. This is the idea of *tai du* or fetal toxins.

Fetal toxins are transferred from the parents to the child in one of two ways. First, they may be passed from either parent to the child at the moment of conception. In this case, the toxicity is due to an unresolved warm disease as discussed above. This is seen as inherited toxicity from a retained or latent hot evil harbored in the parents' blood or *jing*. Second, fetal toxins may develop during gestation due to heat generated internally by the mother from faulty diet or lifestyle.

The consequences of fetal toxins usually manifest as warm diseases during early childhood, such as measles, chicken pox or other pox diseases, scarlatina, and even idiopathic staphylococcus infections of a joint.

In Chinese medicine, it is believed that diseases such as measles or poxes in children should be allowed to run their natural course as much as possible and that skin rashes from such diseases should not be suppressed. If a child can tolerate the disease with little intervention, much of the fetal toxins will then be discharged from the child's body, making him or her a healthier human being.

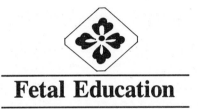

Fetal Education

I n recent years, Western science has established the fact that a fetus in utero is very much aware of sound, light, and the things going on near or around its mother's body. Additionally, women are advised to avoid ingesting alcohol, recreational or unneeded over-the-counter drugs, cigarettes, or other substances that could harm the growing fetus.

While in agreement with all this, the Chinese medical classics also say that a child is strongly influenced by its mother's activities and her mental-emotional state during pregnancy. As we saw in the chapter above on the classical theory of development in utero, the mother is encouraged to do or to avoid a variety of activities and foods to improve her coming child's health and disposition. This idea of being able to influence the child via the mother's behavior, thoughts, and activities is called fetal education. It is an important idea in Chinese medicine with considerable medical literature over the centuries to support it. Fetal education is still promulgated in People's Republic of China today.

The following are several things traditionally to be avoided from the discovery of pregnancy until parturition, or birth: sex; violent action; not sleeping at night; sleeping in the afternoon; forcefully tightening the abdominal muscles; spicy hot, acrid, or heavy food; anything causing constipation; purgatives; emetics; enemas or any medical treatment causing the loss of blood.[1]

---

[1]   *Ambrosia Heart Tantra*, Vol. 1, commentary & translation by Donden & Kelsang, Dharamsala, H.P. India, 1977, p. 55

It is, or was, believed that a woman should practice charity, prayer and contemplation, and meritorious activities as much as possible. She should read uplifting books, stories of saints and sages, hear lectures by learned and cultured persons, and surround herself with beauty and pleasant things. She should avoid ugly scenes, erotic music, and pornographic books. One book, *Admonitions to Ladies*, puts it this way:

> A pregnant woman carries with her the finest piece of jade (*i.e.*, the baby). She should enjoy all things, look at fine pictures, and be attended by handsome servants.[2]

How are we to understand these advisements and how are we to translate them to late 20th century in the West?

First, let us return to Chinese medical theory. In Chinese medicine the body and mind are inseparable, each affecting the other seamlessly. In the chapter on theory above, it was discussed that the spirit or mind resides in the heart. Further, it was said that the heart and uterus are very closely connected by the *chong mai* or *bao mai*. Therefore, anything that influences a woman's mind or spirit affects the heart and can, via these internal channels, also greatly affect the fetus in utero. We have only to think about how strongly a woman can be affected emotionally at different times during her menstrual cycle or how a violent emotional shock can alter the regularity of the menses, to see the importance of the connection between the heart and uterus. Based upon this, classical Chinese physicians felt that if the woman's emotional experiences during pregnancy were pleasant and uplifting, this would have a positive effect on the development of the child and *vice versa*.

---

[2]   As quoted in the *Ambrosia Heart Tantra, op. cit.,* p. 55

Second, if one remembers the importance of family in Asian cultures, it is easy to understand why children were and are considered very precious. They represent the future of the family and the social and eternal security of the parents and grandparents. As such, they are to be protected as well as possible, educated properly, and taught devotion to the family in all things, even before birth. Further, in most Asian cultures, life is not necessarily about the pursuit of pleasure as it often is in the West. Devotion and duty to the larger group (family, clan, community, political cause) are more important than the individual's private needs. Considering this, it is a small thing for the mother to forego gratification of sensual pleasures for a few months in order to ensure the continuity and well being of the child and, thereby, the family and society.

The proscription of sex during pregnancy may seem particularly difficult to modern Western parents. It is advised against partly because of the actual physical discomfort it can cause the fetus, which is described in great detail in Oriental texts, and partly to avoid arousing passions and desires in the fetus. This might create a tendency in the child to be sexually lascivious or overactive in later life. Again it is necessary to stress the idea that, traditionally in Asian cultures, personal, transient pleasures are less important than future consequences for the well being of the child, the family, and the society.

Whether or how much of these ideas about fetal education to accept must be up to the parents, the mother in particular. Classically, there is a whole genre of books devoted to this subject, but the essence of the teaching is summed up in the words of the famous scholar Yuan Seng:

Prenatal education before birth; protection and education after birth.[3]

3   Chen, Chan-yuen, "Medical Commentary on Ancient China," *Oriental Healing Arts Institute Bulletin,* Los Angeles, Jan. 1982, Vol. 7, No. 1, p. 17

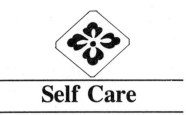

Self Care

M ost pregnant women know the importance of taking the best possible care of themselves during this time. If that were not common knowledge, no one would buy or read this book! However, Chinese medicine has its own approach to self care methods as well as a few new ideas to add to those more commonly discussed. We will discuss each in this chapter.

Diet

During gestation it is, of course, very important that a woman eat a nourishing and well-balanced diet. Since the fetus is feeding on the mother's blood, it is especially important that her diet be specifically designed to promote blood production both for herself and the baby. For the most part, this means supporting the spleen, which is responsible for the day to day production of qi and blood from the purest part of what we eat. Supporting the spleen through diet is done by eating mostly warm, nourishing foods, and fewer cold and raw ones. Pregnancy is not a time for fasting or worrying about the discharge of toxins from the body. In fact, after delivery a woman undergoes one of the most efficient discharges of toxins that she will ever experience.

Where diet is concerned, boosting, supporting, and nourishing are usually more important, than purging or eliminating during pregnancy. Small amounts of animal protein, especially included in vegetable soups, broths, or stews will help to build blood. So will yellow vegetables such as carrots and winter squashes. Oriental foods such as mochi, amasake, sweet rice, litchi, and longans have been used to nourish the blood with time-tested results. However, a woman need not resort to Oriental or exotic foods to get needed blood building nourishment. A sensible diet largely consisting of cooked food, mostly vegetables, grains, and a small amount of meats, is quite adequate. Fruits may be eaten in small quantities. However, an excess of juices, especially citrus juices, will douse the natural or righteous heat of the stomach. This has the effect of slowing digestion and creating excess dampness in the body. This can cause fatigue, qi stagnation, and excessive weight gain.

Food must be warmed up to body temperature before the stomach and spleen can transform it into qi and blood. That is why eating mostly warm, cooked foods, and fewer raw, iced, or chilled foods is very important. Chilled and raw foods require more work from the spleen and stomach, and leaves less energy for them from which to create qi and blood.

Food should also be fresh and freshly prepared as much as possible. This is because fresh foods have more qi, and qi is required to create blood. Foods that have been cooked, refrigerated, and then reheated over several days lack qi — in Chinese they are called "wrecked food." Ideally food should be eaten within 24 hours of being cooked.

Many pregnant women ask whether they are getting enough vitamins, calcium, and/or protein from their diets, especially if they are strict vegetarians. It is my experience as a practitioner and as a mother that pregnant women do better if they consume at least a small amount of animal protein. It is true that protein deficiency is quite rare in Americans or people of other similarly well-fed cultures. However, from the point of view of Chinese medicine, it is easier to make more blood from well cooked, easily digested animal foods, than solely from vegetable sources. By small amounts, I mean 2-3 ounces, perhaps 3 or 4 times per week. This can be in the form of soups, broths, or stews which make meat easier to digest and which may be more palatable to women for whom meat is not normally part of their diet. Pork, beef, buffalo, venison, elk, or mutton are all fine. Eggs are also a very nutritious food and can be included in the diet on a regular basis. Fish and fowl are also good, but one should be careful that chicken does not become the main form of animal protein in the diet. This is because chicken's nature is quite hot. This means that, when ingested too often, it can produce excessive heat in the body. This warning goes back to our earlier discussion of warm or hot diseases and their relationship to fetal toxins. It is better to eat a variety of meats, taking each kind no more than once per week.

Also, it is best to try to find a hormone- and antibiotic-free source of eggs, chicken, and meat in general. It is unclear what effect these substances might have on a developing fetus. We do know, however, that such additives are not good for us and so are best avoided as much as possible.

Dairy products may be eaten in moderation as well, but 2-3 servings per day, as suggested by Western nutritionists, are way too much from the point of view of Chinese medicine. Dairy products are very damp, and cold dairy products are even more damp than cooked ones. If a woman develops any symptoms such as a runny nose, chest congestion, excessive vaginal discharge, or if she is gaining too much weight, dairy products should be cut back or cut out temporarily. If calcium or mineral ingestion is a worry, I suggest that women take a good prenatal vitamin/mineral supplement of which there are many good ones on the market. Also, leafy, green vegetables, fish, nuts, meat, and sea vegetables are all good sources of calcium and other minerals and are less likely to produce excess dampness in the body.

It is common for women to experience all sorts of cravings, especially during the early stages of the pregnancy. When a craving arises, it should be gratified initially with a very small amount of the desired food. If just one or two bites satisfy the craving, that is all one should eat. However, one should take those one or two bites even if one does not ordinarily eat this food or consider it healthy. If not satisfied by only a small amount, it is probably an inappropriate craving on the part of the mother. These should not be indulged in the case of junk foods, or indulged with caution if the food is a healthy one. Oriental texts stress the importance of satisfying the child's cravings during pregnancy, even urging the mother to eat otherwise strange, revolting, or non-nutritious substances, if only a very small amount.[4]

In terms of food and weight gain, it is thought that the woman should gain sufficient weight to have a reserve of blood after the child is born so that she is not depleted to the point of blood vacuity. She will need still more blood after the birth since milk is made from blood. On the other hand, excessive weight gain will lead to an accumulation of dampness in the body. This can cause a variety of other complications both during pregnancy and after the child is born. Western medical texts advise 24-40 lbs. as normal. More than 40 lbs. is likely to lead to permanent overweight in the mother. Although Chinese texts do not give specific numbers, these numbers seem about right depending upon the size of the woman. Some Chinese doctors also say that a healthy mother should take nine months to lose the weight that she gained during the nine months of pregnancy. Too fast a weight loss after pregnancy can be as detrimental to the health as too much of a weight gain during pregnancy. Again, Chinese medicine stresses moderation and the doctrine of the mean.

Exercise

If food is yin (substance), then exercise is the yang (function) which balances it. While classic Chinese medical texts forbid strenuous physical exercise during pregnancy, it must be remembered that a

---

[4]   "Medical Commentary In Ancient China", *op. cit.*, p. 52

woman living in a traditional culture, even a member of the aristocracy, would very likely get plenty of exercise in the normal course of her life. In pretechnological societies, even the rich needed to do far more physical labor for themselves than most poor in late 20th century Western societies.

Regular exercise does many important things for a pregnant woman. Most of the health problems that arise during pregnancy are due to one of two disease mechanisms: qi and blood vacuity or qi stagnation and blood stasis. Exercise is beneficial in preventing or ameliorating both of these.

First, just as one must often spend money to make money, the movement of qi and blood through exercise catalyzes the body to create more qi and blood by improving spleen and stomach function. The role of spleen and stomach in relationship to the production of qi and blood has been discussed in the first chapter on Chinese medical theory. However, to review, it is the job of the spleen and stomach to create qi and blood from the pure part of the food and liquids that we digest. Moderate, regular exercise improves this function.

Second, exercise helps rid the body of stagnation by keeping everything in motion internally. People will often say that they blow off steam and stress by a good workout at the gym or a fast game of racketball. This is literally true. Stress creates pathological heat in the body. When heat builds internally and has no way to be released, it can cause a variety of health problems. It is like a pressure cooker with too much pressure inside. Exercise helps release this pressure, like opening the release valve on the top of the cooker.

This is very important for the health of the liver which, as was described in the introductory chapter on theory, is responsible for the smooth, even flow of qi through the body. The liver is sometimes called the "temperamental organ." This means that it is the organ most adversely affected by the stresses and frustrations of modern life. If qi becomes stagnant or stuck, the liver is usually involved. Stagnant liver qi plays a part in many health problems that may attend pregnancy and labor, including morning sickness and difficult labor. Therefore, exercise is vital for the health of the liver during pregnancy and, actually, at all times in our life.

Third, combined with dietary regulation, exercise is the best defense against the accumulation of dampness in the body. Movement stimulates the transportation and transformation of dampness and phlegm that might otherwise accumulate as fat.

Fourth, moderate exercise strengthens the lungs and heart and helps keep the bowels open. The lungs are responsible for the circulation of qi, the health of the skin and hair, and the proper descension and dispersion of fluids in the body. The heart's role in sending blood to the uterus and circulating it throughout the body has already been discussed above. And, since constipation is a common problem during pregnancy, open, healthy bowels are also important. Therefore, we can see that exercise is really vital for the health of most of the organs and bowels in the body.

Finally, women who exercise regularly during pregnancy statistically have easier and shorter labors. Labor is called labor because it is hard work. A woman can literally think of her prenatal exercise as a training regime for this one event — her own, personal Olympic event.

Exercise during pregnancy, however, should have some limitations. Sky diving, bungee jumping, technical climbing, and other sports with a high degree of danger may not be the best choices. While a very athletic woman may keep up a good deal of her regular exercise routine until quite late in the pregnancy, the best all around exercises for pregnancy are probably walking, swimming, stretching, and other mildly aerobic activities. Most cities and towns have special yoga or aerobics classes for pregnant women. These can be very good for women who do not already have an exercise program.

While she is huffing and puffing, a mother should keep in mind that she is doing this for herself as well as her baby. Anything that naturally makes labor shorter and easier is worth the time and effort. It is as simple as that.

Quiet Time

We live in a time when most women must work outside the home in order for their family to have a modestly comfortable life style. Many women are mothers, cooks and housekeepers, and volunteers as well. When we work too hard, juggling our various hats, stress begins to take its toll. While rest and relaxation is vital for all of us, it is absolutely crucial for a mother-to-be. Time to read a book, make a flower arrangement, putter around the house, or just sit and daydream creates space and relaxes the mind. This need not necessarily be a formal relaxation or meditation practice, but work must be balanced by adequate rest and relaxation or what I like to call "down time." Most of the women I know do not get enough of this in their lives. For pregnant women it is even more important to have time for quiet reflection, a time when demands on her energy and attention are, at least temporarily, relieved.

For women who have a hard time doing this regularly, I strongly suggest the use of relaxation tapes. These are relatively inexpensive and are widely available at book, new age, or health food stores. Your health care practitioner can probably suggest some for you. Such tapes are easy to use, and quite effective in helping a person achieve both mental and physical relaxation if used on a regular basis. For people who lack the discipline to relax in any other way, tapes may be quite helpful. For more detail on the clinical usefulness of relaxation tapes, the reader may want to see my book *Second Spring: A Guide to Healthy Menopause Through Traditional Chinese Medicine*, which has an entire chapter dedicated to this subject.

Self Massage

Self-massage can have several useful effects for a pregnant woman. First, it is a way to take time out for herself, to pay attention to herself. Second, it helps to move the qi and blood and prevent stagnation. Third, it helps keep the skin supple and moist, allowing it to stretch more easily, especially the belly and perineum. Fourth, vigorous massage of the nipples (dry-brushing) can help prepare them for nursing.

Self-massage can take several forms. When I was pregnant, I practiced two types of massage: dry-brushing all over and oil massage of my abdomen and perineal areas to prevent stretch marks. I found both to be effective.

Dry-brushing is a form of massage done with a stiff bristle brush attached to a long handle, allowing one to reach down the back. It is most often suggested to be done first thing in the morning all over the body except the external genitalia. It can be effective for toughening up the nipples, which often become sore during the first week or two of nursing. According to Chinese medicine, this type of stimulation of the skin helps to circulate the qi in the most superficial of the body channels and increases blood flow in the skin. It is helpful in preventing stagnation and in keeping the skin well nourished. This is important when one considers how much the skin of the abdomen and breasts must stretch during pregnancy. Dry-brushing also helps to shed dead skin cells, allowing the skin to breathe, and to grow new cells more efficiently.

While oil massage may provide some nutrients to the skin, healthy skin is truly a reflection of internal health and vitality. Nevertheless, most midwives suggest that a woman apply creams or oils to the perineum regularly during the later stages of pregnancy to help it stretch during delivery. I myself followed this advice and was lucky enough not to require an episiotomy during my son's birth.

Other useful forms of self-massage may include reflexology, a type of foot massage by which one can influence all the other parts of the body, and *dao yin* or *do in*, which is self-massage that one does all over the body with pressing, tapping, or rubbing. There are several books out on both these subjects (see Suggested Reading at the back of this book). It is best to be gentle when doing any form of self-massage. The idea is to provide mild stimulation to the skin, organs, and tissues of the body.

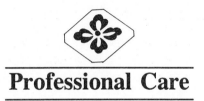

Professional Care

A pregnant woman may seek professional care for both preventive and remedial purposes. Practitioners of Chinese medicine have a lot to offer in either or both areas, although in Chinese medicine prevention is always emphasized. First, however, let us discuss a type of preventive care that may or may not be done by a Chinese medical practitioner.

Massage

The massage of pregnant women and newly birthed mothers has become something of a specialty in massage training institutions in the West. Special pads are available which make it possible for a pregnant woman to lie comfortably on a massage practitioner's table in a variety of positions. There are even books available on just this type of massage. If you are pregnant and not receiving massage, I strongly suggest that it become a regular part of your preventive health regime if it is available in your area and if you can afford it. This is especially important in the final trimester when your body may feel large and unwieldy and the skin is being stretched to its limits.

Massage allows a pregnant woman or a new mother the time and space to rest, relax, and be nurtured by caring hands. The mother who feels nurtured herself is better able to nurture her child, both in the womb and newly born. That alone is enough of a reason to receive massage during the childbearing year, but there are others as well.

By relieving stress, massage is relaxing to the liver, the importance of which has been discussed already. It is also said in Chinese medicine that the sinews or connective tissue are related to the liver. Relaxing and releasing the connective tissue through massage has a direct, positive effect on the health of the liver.

Massage also increases the flow of blood and qi to the four limbs, reducing the possibility of stagnation. During the third trimester of pregnancy this is even more needed because the fetus is so large as to make proper flow of blood and qi more difficult. For many women, movement and exercise, which would help prevent qi and blood stagnation, become more limited as the weeks go by. While massage is not a total replacement for exercise, it can help prevent some problems that lack of exercise is likely to create.

Massage helps circulate qi, blood, and body fluids in the skin. If a woman is experiencing edema in the ankles and feet during the final weeks of pregnancy, massage can help eliminate this. Also, the emollient effect of the oils or creams nourishes the skin and helps it to stay supple and soft.

During labor, massage can be used to help reduce the discomfort of contractions and to gently stretch the perineum so that an episiotomy is unnecessary.

During the postpartum months, massage does all the same things. Perhaps just the feeling that someone is taking care of you for a little while is the most important feeling of all.

Acupuncture/Moxibustion

There has been a great deal of confusion about the use of acupuncture during pregnancy. Some acupuncture texts say that it is not advised, but not prohibited. Other books say merely that it is not the modality of choice during pregnancy, and herbal medicine is more advisable.

While it is not advisable to use acupuncture frivolously during pregnancy, the truth is that acupuncture and moxibustion can be very useful for a variety of problems that may arise during this time. If done by a trained practitioner, it is not dangerous. There are certain points which one is advised not to needle during pregnancy, but all acupuncturists who have been properly trained should be well aware of these. While herbal medicine may generally be a better choice for problems that arise during pregnancy, there are some gestational problems for which acupuncture is actually a better choice than herbs.

Morning sickness is a good example of this. That is because, for women who are experiencing nausea, the smell and taste of Chinese herbal medicine may be intolerable. They may vomit merely from the smell of it or be unable to get it down. Acupuncture, on the other hand, can work very well to eliminate their discomfort in only a few treatments. There are also other problems during pregnancy that respond positively to acupuncture, especially those that require forceful, immediate treatment, such as preeclampsia. Acupuncture may also be used to hasten or initiate labor that is slowed or delayed, or to reduce the discomfort of contractions.

Moxibustion, which is the burning of mugwort, *Folium Artemesiae (Ai Ye)*, on, over, under, or around certain acupoints on the body, may also be used to good effect in many situations. While acupuncture can only manipulate qi that is already available in the body, moxibustion (moxa) is believed to be able to add qi to the body. For women who have problems during pregnancy due to depletion or vacuity of qi and blood, moxibustion may be quite effective, especially if herbal medicine is not available.

Moxa is also the treatment of choice for malposition of the fetus or breech presentation. During the final month of pregnancy it can be used on a specific point to try to turn the fetus. However, this technique is more effective for a transverse as opposed to a truly breech presentation. In either case, the sooner such treatments are begun, the more effective they are.

From all this we can see that acupuncture and moxibustion are useful modalities which can be safe and effective in solving many problems that commonly arise during pregnancy.

Chinese Herbal Medicine

Although acupuncture is better known in the West, herbal medicine is the main modality of Chinese medicine. The word herbal is somewhat of a misnomer since Chinese doctors prescribe vegetable, animal, and mineral medicinals. When prescribed professionally, these are usually combined in multi-ingredient formulas which are then decocted and drunk as a very strong tea several times per day.

Such Chinese herbal decoctions are different from Western folk herbal remedies. First, the amount of raw materials per dose is usually larger. Secondly, most of the ingredients are roots and twigs as opposed to leaves and flowers and are, therefore, stronger for that reason as well. Third, most of the formulas that Chinese doctors prescribe have been used in clinical practice for hundreds and, in many cases, even thousands of years. Thus, they have been well tested in clinical practice. Fourth, they are prescribed according to a professional, albeit Chinese, differential diagnosis. And fifth, they are modified to fit the individual patient as precisely as possible. Because of this, Chinese herbal formulas have no side effects when prescribed by a well-trained and experienced practitioner.

The practice of prescribing and combining the 5-600 main medicinals in the traditional Chinese pharmacopeia is a high art and takes years to truly master. However, it is also one of the world's most effective medical systems. There are formulas to treat every condition that might arise during pregnancy, delivery, and postpartum. Because this medicine is strong, its effects are quick-acting. Yet because the ingredients are natural and blended with such care and precision, there are no side effects and very little chance of doctor-induced reactions. And, unlike modern Western medicine which is mainly prescribed on the basis of a disease diagnosis - every patient with the same disease getting the same medication - traditional Chinese practitioners mainly prescribe on the basis of each individual patient's total pattern.

In a recently released Chinese medical textbook, *Path of Pregnancy, Vol. I: A Handbook of Traditional Chinese Gestational & Birthing Diseases*, there are close to 30 conditions that may crop up during pregnancy and delivery for which Chinese herbal formulas are given. Under each of these diseases or conditions, there are then several individual patterns with their own appropriate formulas. In a companion volume concerning postpartum care and recuperation, *Path of Pregnancy, Vol. II: A Handbook of Traditional Chinese Postpartum Diseases,* there are more than another 30 diseases and conditions addressed by Chinese herbal medicine.

The following chapters describe some of the diseases and conditions encountered during pregnancy, delivery, and postpartum that Chinese medicine addresses. For each and every one of these, there are safe and effective, nontoxic and noniatrogenic Chinese herbal therapy. By this, I do not mean to imply that Chinese herbal medicine is sufficient to replace modern Western medicine. It is not. However, because of the high potential for side effects and medicine-induced reactions with modern Western pharmaceuticals, it is my opinion that, in many cases, Chinese herbal medicine should be tried first in a graduated series of responses. If it does not work, then the patient can move on to a stronger, more aggressive Western therapy. However, to me it makes sense to first try a more holistic, safer, and often less expensive approach.

Problems During Pregnancy

Diagnosis & Treatment in Chinese Medicine

A t the beginning of this book, in the chapter on Chinese medical theory, several ideas about the differences between traditional Chinese medicine and Western biomedical medicine were discussed. However, before we can present specific problems during pregnancy and how they are treated by Chinese medicine, another difference between the two medical systems must be introduced.

Western medical diagnosis and treatment are based upon named diseases or disease categories which are seen to be caused by specific pathogens or internal biochemical imbalances. In Chinese, this type of categorization of human dysfunction according to named diseases is called *bian bing* diagnosis, or diagnosis according to a discrimination of diseases. Western medicine uses this type of diagnosis. All patients diagnosed with the same disease in this type of medical system are typically prescribed the same medicine or type of medicine.

B*ian bing* diagnosis also exists in Chinese medicine and historically there were doctors who dispensed their therapies solely on the basis of disease diagnosis. Today, however, it is typically combined with another style of diagnosis and treatment as well, called *bian zheng lun zhi*, or diagnosis and treatment according to the discrimination of patterns (of disharmony). Disease (*bing*) and pattern (*zheng*) are not the same. A pattern of disharmony is the total constellation of the signs and symptoms of an individual patient. A disease, however, is usually defined by a much narrower group of signs and symptoms. Two patients having the same disease usually share certain key signs and symptoms. Additionally, they may each display other different symptoms which may or may not be related to that disease. In Chinese medicine, while these two patients may have the same disease (*bing*), they may each have a different pattern (*zheng*) and should therefore receive different treatment. This is one explanation of why a medicine may work very well for one patient with a named disease, but not work at all in another or, even worse, cause severe side effects. Those two patients may have the same disease (*bing*), but not the same pattern (*zheng*) within that disease category. The importance of Chinese medicine pattern diagnosis is, therefore, that it allows individualized, specific treatment based upon the whole person. Typically in China, a person will receive both a pattern and a disease diagnosis. If done correctly, this is more effective than disease diagnosis alone and prevents side effects from treatment. Ridding a symptom in one part of the body only to cause another symptom in another part is not considered acceptable in Chinese medicine since the organism is seen as a single, integrated unit.

To make this clearer, let's again use the example of morning sickness. In Chinese medicine, morning sickness is called "nausea and vomiting during pregnancy." That is the *bing* or named disease category. However, if you talk to 3 or 4 women who have morning sickness, you will quickly see that each has a different experience of this condition with a different set of signs and symptoms. In Chinese medicine, there are 5 main patterns of disharmony which account for nausea and vomiting during pregnancy (morning sickness). These are:

1. Spleen/stomach vacuity weakness
2. Phlegm dampness obstruction and stagnation
3. Liver invading stomach
4. Liver depression transforming into heat
5. Qi & yin dual vacuity

Each of these 5 patterns of disharmony has its own distinguishing signs, symptoms, tongue and pulse signs. Each also requires its own, individual treatment plan, be that with herbal medicine or acupuncture if the patient is to be treated effectively and without side effects. In real life patients, there may be more than one pattern of disharmony manifesting simultaneously in the same patient. Treatment must, therefore, be adjusted to account for both or all of the concurrent patterns. If the pattern (*zheng*) diagnosis and subsequent treatment are skillful, the disease (*bing*) will be dealt with effectively and without complications.

Named Disease Categories During Pregnancy in Traditional Chinese Medicine

The traditional *tai qian bing* or gestational diseases include nausea and vomiting, abdominal pain, restless fetal movement, vaginal bleeding, miscarriage, habitual miscarriage, edema, diarrhea, dysentery, cough, loss of voice, urinary problems, malaria-like disease, so-called fetal epilepsy, dizziness, insanity, vexation, and dysphoria. To these, modern Chinese medicine has added hypertension, preeclampsia, eclampsia, ectopic pregnancy, hydatidiform mole, and chorioadenoma. However, these are but modern names which cover aspects of traditional diseases. For instance, ectopic pregnancy as a modern disease category is associated with abdominal pain, and so-called fetal epilepsy is eclampsia. Below is a list of complaints during pregnancy as they are described by Chinese medicine, with details about the most important ones.

Nausea & vomiting during pregnancy (morning sickness)

No matter which of the 5 patterns of disharmony listed above account for the nausea and vomiting, nausea *per se* has to do with a disharmony of the stomach. Stomach qi is supposed to go down. In nausea and vomiting the qi counterflows (flows in the wrong direction) upward. If the proper pattern can be determined, the proper flow of qi can be restored by either acupuncture and/or herbal medicine.

As discussed above, acupuncture is often an effective choice for this problem. If the case is very serious, it may need to be done daily, with treatments lasting as long as 1 hour. Magnets or magnet bracelets may be used to treat minor nausea or to continue therapy between scheduled acupuncture treatments. It should also be remembered that in cases where a woman has progesterone insufficiency or a history of infertility or habitual miscarriage, morning sickness may be seen as a good sign. This is because it indicates healthy ovarian function at least *vis à vis* progesterone.

Abdominal pain during pregnancy

Pain in the lower abdomen during pregnancy can suggest an impending miscarriage. While Chinese medical therapy can treat this condition effectively, it is important for a woman to be assured that the treatment will not prevent a miscarriage in cases of a blighted ovum or abnormal fetus. The treatment is only effective for stopping miscarriage due to an imbalance or deficiency in the mother. Pain in the abdomen during pregnancy should be treated with Chinese herbal medicine and/or acupuncture as soon as it arises.

Ectopic pregnancy

Ectopic pregnancy refers to the condition when the fetus implants outside the main cavity of the uterus. In this case, the fetus may erroneously attach to the walls of the fallopian tubes, the ovaries, or even in the abdominal cavity.

This condition begins as abdominal pain, but usually becomes severe quite quickly. This is a surgical condition, even in China. Its modern Western treatment should not be delayed.

In China today, there are herbal protocols which are being used to treat ectopic pregnancy in those who, for various reasons, cannot undergo surgery. These consist of two steps. The first formula, given for several days kills the fetus, while the second step ensures that the aborted conceptus is expelled.

Hydatidiform mole

This is another condition better suited for Western medical treatment since it can be associated with malignancy. It is typically the end stage of a degenerating pregnancy in which the cells have undergone varying amounts of abnormal proliferation. These cells may be either benign or cancerous in nature and are called moles because *mola* means mass. This condition is most commonly seen in older women and may be accompanied by a variety of other symptoms including bleeding and infection.

Miscarriage or threatened abortion

In Chinese medicine, this condition has several stages and levels of severity and thus several possible disease names: fetal leakage, restless stirring of the fetus, falling fetus, and small birth. Within each of these disease categories there are several possible patterns of disharmony as discussed above.

There are 5 basic mechanisms associated with miscarriage according to traditional Chinese medicine. The first is kidney vacuity. It is kidney qi that consolidates the fetus and astringes the anal and vaginal orifices. If, due to congenital weakness and insufficiency, age, chronic disease, or extreme and/or prolonged taxation, the internal channels become vacuous and empty, the fetus may not be consolidated and secured in place.

Secondly, if food and drink are not well regulated, if one works too hard, or suffers from excessive worry and anxiety, the spleen and stomach may become vacuous and weak. A strong spleen is required to restrain and hold up the abdominal contents including the uterus with the fetus inside.

Third, mental agitation and emotional frustration, envy, anger, or excessive jealousy may all give rise internally to depressive fire. This heat may cause the blood to "boil over" and flow recklessly downward and the fetus may have no place on which to rest and rely.

Fourth, it is possible also for blood stasis to force the blood outside its normal pathways thus causing bleeding or what is called fetal leakage.

And fifth, external injury, such as falling from a height, being hit or struck, or sustaining a sprain or strain may damage and injure the *chong mai* and other internal channels.

Chinese medicine can treat all these disease categories effectively if treatment is sought in time and if treatment is aggressive. Even if a woman passes a large amount of blood and even with clots, she should not automatically think that she has miscarried until a pregnancy test can be done, followed by a gynecological exam and/or ultrasonography.

Slippery fetus (habitual miscarriage)

This describes a situation of 3 or more repeated miscarriages. It is commonly encountered in women with difficulty in getting pregnant and most often in women in their 30s and 40s. Insufficient qi and kidney emptiness are usually the causes. Historically, Chinese doctors have suggested that a woman take herbal medicine for 6 months or so before again attempting to get pregnant. Each successive miscarriage causes further injury to the kidneys, also causing or aggravating stagnant blood in the uterus. This condition is often due to constitutional weakness or debility and decline due to the aging process, aggravated by emotional stress, overwork, and poor diet.

Because Western doctors inform their patients that most miscarriages are due to genetic malformation of the fetus and its subsequent inviability, many Western women are confused about taking Chinese medicine to forestall a threatened abortion. The Chinese medical literature suggests that every threatening miscarriage should be treated according to a pattern discrimination diagnosis since there are many other factors besides malformation of the fetus that can cause a spontaneous abortion. Chinese medical literature suggests that if the fetus is genetically inviable, no amount of Chinese herbs are going to save it and continue the pregnancy. In that case, the issue is a disease of the fetus. Here we are talking about the mother's disease or condition. While this a decision that a woman must make for herself, I know of no case where treatment by Chinese medicine for threatened miscarriage has resulted in the birth of a malformed baby.

Incompetent cervix or late term spontaneous miscarriage

During the last weeks of the second trimester or the first weeks of the last trimester, some women will spontaneously abort due to an incompetent cervix. This means that the cervix is too weak to hold in the fetus which has now grown in size and weight. Modern Western medicine treats this condition by sewing the cervix together like the strings of a purse. However, this is only done at the start of the second pregnancy, after the woman has already lost one baby due to this condition. In a prima para (woman pregnant for the first time), all Western medicine can offer is to tell the woman to lie in bed for the rest of the pregnancy. In any case, the woman still usually delivers prematurely.

According to Bob Flaws, a well-known TCM gynecology specialist, the TCM cause of this condition is typically spleen qi vacuity. In this case, the spleen qi, which is responsible for holding up the abdominal contents, is too weak to hold up the ever-growing, heavier and heavier fetus. Dr. Flaws has had success in forestalling several miscarriages in late stage women suffering from incompetent cervices. He use a combination of Chinese herbal medicinals designed to supplement the center (i.e., the spleen) and boost the qi. This was combined with the use of moxibustion a the crown of the head to raise up the qi which hold up the baby. As in modern Western medicine, it is still important that the woman remain in bed.

Based on Dr. Flaws' experience, it is important that pregnant women with spleen qi vacuity not stand too long, not allow themselves to become too fatigued, and that they begin taking Chinese herbal medicine to fortify the spleen and boost the qi beginning around the fifth or sixth month of pregnancy when their abdomens become markedly distended. Since the *Nei Jing* states that the spleen naturally begins to weaken at 35 years of age, women in their midd-30s and older should be screened for this condition and be treated preventively.

Fetus declines, does not grow

This is due to lack of nourishment to the fetus in turn due to insufficient qi and blood. This may be due to congenital insufficiency, chronic disease, age, weakness of the spleen and stomach, or overwork and overtaxation. Happily, there are Chinese herbal formulas for the treatment of this condition which supplement the qi and nourish the blood.

Dead fetus does not descend

This is a condition that is unlikely to be seen by a practitioner of Chinese medicine. If suspected, it should be referred to a practitioner of Western medicine.

Edema during pregnancy (water swelling)

In Chinese medicine, body fluids are controlled by three organs, the kidneys, spleen, and lungs. If water builds up in tissues where it is not supposed to be, it is always due to some problem with one or more of these organs. The problem is either an insufficiency of qi which then cannot transform and move the liquids adequately, or stagnation of qi which then leads to stagnation of dampness. Whether edema manifests in the face, hands, or feet and lower legs, there are effective Chinese herbal formulas to treat this.

Diarrhea during pregnancy

Diarrhea at any time is usually due to either weakness of or cold injury to the spleen or by dampness and heat in the bowels. While the causes during pregnancy are the same, it is most urgent that the diarrhea be stopped as soon as possible because diarrhea indicates that digestion is impaired. A woman with impaired digestion is unable to create the large amounts of qi, blood, and *jing* necessary to nourish herself and her child during pregnancy. Chinese herbal medicine is particularly effective for stopping diarrhea. Usually, practitioners will also give advice about dietary changes and prohibitions.

Cough during pregnancy

This problem is usually due to one of two pathoconditions. The spleen may be weak and not producing enough qi to properly transform fluids which then build up and lodge in the lungs. In this case, the cough will most likely produce phlegm. On the other hand, the entire yin of the body (substance: blood, fluids, *jing*) may be empty and vacuous during pregnancy due to increased demands on the blood. If this happens, the body's yang (function: qi, warmth, movement) is not balanced and held down where it belongs. Yang is warm in nature. If not balanced by adequate yin, it rises up into the upper part of the body. In this situation it leads to a cough that will usually not produce phlegm. In both cases, Chinese herbal medicine can be effective. If due to faulty diet and spleen dampness, proper diet is extremely important. If due to yin vacuity, Chinese medicine can usually benefit the cough. In some cases, however, the cough will not disappear totally until after delivery.

61

Child aphonia (loss of voice during pregnancy)

Laryngitis or hoarseness during pregnancy usually occurs in the later stages of pregnancy and is due to the largeness of the fetus cutting off the connection between the lungs and kidneys. In such cases, the kidneys are often weak already and the pregnancy merely adds a further strain on them. This condition, like yin vacuity cough above, can be benefitted by Chinese herbal medicine but may not be cured until after delivery, when it spontaneously disappears.

Child strangury (urinary difficulties during pregnancy)

Urinary problems during pregnancy are common. These may include frequent or urgent urination, feelings of incompleteness after urination, dribbling between urination, burning sensations when urinating, or difficulty urinating. These difficulties may be at least partially due to the position of the bladder, which is being squeezed or constrained more and more as the fetus grows larger. Furthermore, in Chinese medicine, proper bladder function is a result of healthy kidney qi. During pregnancy the kidneys are under a great deal more stress than usual, which may lead to bladder symptoms. Finally, if a woman does not regulate her diet properly, this may be complicated by dampness and heat becoming lodged in the bladder. Such bladder and urinary problems typically respond to Chinese herbal medicine.

Fetal epilepsy (preeclampsia, eclampsia, high blood pressure during pregnancy, albuminuria)

Fetal epilepsy is merely an ancient term for the Western medical conditions preeclampsia and eclampsia. It is also referred to in modern Chinese texts as albuminuria (excessive proteins in the urine) or high blood pressure during pregnancy. These conditions usually arise late in pregnancy and are progressive in nature. Therefore, treatment must be begun in the earliest stages to be successful in forestalling further development. Chinese herbal medicine and acupuncture can be very effective in preeclampsia, and can prevent the condition from devolving into a life-threatening emergency. However, a woman must be very carefully monitored by both her Chinese and Western medical practitioner. If the condition is not responding to therapy she must be sent to the emergency room to seek Western medical care immediately.

Mild preeclampsia is characterized by borderline high blood pressure, edema or swelling in the face and limbs, and high levels of protein in the urine. If these conditions are not checked, the woman may develop full-fledged eclampsia, very high blood pressure, coma, and/or convulsions. The primary Western medical treatment for both preeclampsia and eclampsia is induced delivery. This can mean a premature birth and usually a Caesarean section.

The Chinese medical diagnosis of this condition is somewhat complex for a book of this type. It usually involves imbalances in several organs and substances simultaneously. Its diagnosis and treatment, however, are quite thoroughly described in the Chinese clinical literature existing in English. A woman who suspects that she may have preeclampsia should not hesitate to seek Chinese medical treatment as long as she is also being monitored by a Western physician.

Other conditions during pregnancy

Chinese medicine also describes several other possible diseases during pregnancy that are typically not seen as diseases of pregnancy by Western medicine. These include: cold injury, summerheat strike, dampness strike (all varieties of the flu or common cold), malarial disease, acute gastroenteritis, acid regurgitation, headache, and various conditions of the eyes, nose, throat, lips, and mouth during pregnancy. All these diseases have pattern diagnosis breakdowns and effective Chinese herbal treatment plans.

Finally, there is yet another category of diseases described by Chinese medicine as arising during pregnancy. These include child vexation, child suspension, fetus forcing up the heart, and child insanity. The symptoms of all these are emotional dysfunction, anxiety, or agitation of the mother, and there are treatments described in the literature to calm these emotional storms. Therefore, women experiencing otherwise undiagnosable psychological distress should see a practitioner of Chinese medicine. Often a course of Chinese herbs can allay the woman's anxiety, agitation, or insomnia.

Conclusion

Because of the sophistication and holism of its diagnosis as described briefly above, Chinese medicine can treat most complaints encountered during pregnancy effectively and inexpensively. These should be corrected as soon as possible so that organ/bowel function is not compromised, resulting in either diminished production of qi and blood or its impaired flow. Thus both the mother's and the fetus' health and survival are guaranteed.

Preparing for Delivery

B y the middle of the third trimester of pregnancy a woman should begin to prepare for labor and delivery. If she has been receiving primary care from a practitioner of Chinese medicine, he or she will probably have discussed this with the mother-to-be already. If one has not yet received Chinese medical care, this would be a good time to seek out a qualified practitioner.

During the eighth month of pregnancy, a woman who is under the care of a practitioner of Chinese medicine will be assessed to decide what needs to be done to help her have a successful labor with the least discomfort and complications. Not every woman will need the same intervention and indeed, a woman who has been receiving good advice and care right along during the pregnancy may not need any intervention at all.

Most often, there are two things that a practitioner of Chinese medicine might wish to do at this point in the pregnancy.

1. Activate the qi and move the blood

If a woman has any tendency to stagnation and stasis in the pelvis, herbs may be prescribed which will help reduce this. Stagnation of qi typically slows the process of labor and stasis of blood usually makes it more painful. Therefore, any treatment that can accomplish the task of reducing these two stagnations will have an effect called *cui sheng*, to hasten or smooth the process of birth. This treatment may be begun during the eighth month.

2. Supplementing qi and nourishing the blood

Pregnancy makes such increased demands on the spleen and kidneys to create qi and blood and to nourish the fetus. Women whose spleens or kidneys are not as strong as necessary may find themselves depleted during the later stages of pregnancy, their qi and/or blood becoming insufficient for their own health. This is more common as a woman gets older and her spleen and kidneys have naturally begun to decline.

It should be noted again that the qi and blood are a yin/yang pair. The qi commands the blood, and one of its functions is to hold the blood within its vessels. If the qi becomes weak during pregnancy and this problem is not redressed successfully, it will be less able to do this job during labor. This can lead to excessive bleeding both during and after the labor, which then may lead to blood vacuity and emptiness. If this happens, postpartum recuperation may be slow and other health problems that require more difficult and long-term care may arise.

It should also be remembered that labor itself requires great amounts of qi, as do the early days and weeks of mothering. Furthermore, breast milk is made from blood. Therefore, insufficient or vacuous qi and blood are better dealt with as much as possible before labor begins. In such cases, Chinese herbs may be prescribed and/or moxibustion may be done to boost or supplement the qi and blood.

Malposition of the Fetus

During the final weeks of pregnancy it may also be discovered that the fetus is malpositioned. Since most Western obstetricians will require a Caesarean section delivery in such cases, it is always best to try to turn the fetus to the normal, head down, position. Many midwives and obstetricians may try a technique called manual version. MDs will only perform this technique in a hospital since it can result in inadvertent rupture of the amniotic sac. In this case, labor must usually be induced within 24 hours or a C-section performed.

Chinese medicine has a technique that can be effective in many cases if begun soon enough during gestation, say the 32nd or 33rd week. This is the technique of using indirect moxibustion on a point on the pregnant woman's feet, 2-3 times per day for 15 to 20 minutes at a time. This technique has been widely used in China, and there are numerous clinical reports corroborating it to be safe and effective. The later in the pregnancy the technique is applied, however, the less likely it is to be effective. Certainly, for women whose babies are not in the correct position, this method is worth trying to avoid a Caesarean birth if possible.

Labor & Delivery

M uch has been written about the humane management of labor. As one might expect, Chinese medicine advocates as little intervention as possible, allowing it to proceed naturally and at its own pace. However, skillful intervention may sometimes be useful, and both acupuncture and herbal medicine may play a role, depending upon what is needed.

Pain Control

Women experience varying levels of discomfort during labor and delivery. While some women find the pain quite overwhelming, others say that it is not a big deal at all. Some women say it feels like strong menstrual cramps, for others like a severe low back-ache.

While there are a variety of Western medical techniques that can be very effective for relieving pain during labor, they have some disadvantages. Pain medication can have the effect of making a woman drowsy or putting her to sleep altogether. However, the birth of a child is an exciting event for most women and definitely not to be missed because of being drugged — not unless really necessary!

Also, use of such pain medication usually means that a woman must lie down and cannot walk, squat, or move around. The first stages of labor are much easier for many women if they can walk, move around, and otherwise change their position frequently. This moving may even help speed the labor along. Furthermore, pain medication can have the effect of slowing labor down and/or depressing normal fetal respiration. If the latter occur, further intervention either with drugs or Caesarean section may be required. Finally, it is known that anything that enters the mother's bloodstream will enter the child's as well, and this includes drugs used during labor and delivery.

The other most common Western medical option for pain relief is the epidural. This is a numbing agent which is injected into the lower spinal cord that numbs the entire nervous system from the waist down. This has the advantage of leaving the woman wide awake, but the disadvantage that she cannot feel anything in her pelvis. Thus, it is difficult for her to feel if she is pushing or not during the second stage of labor and delivery. Epidural injections may also have side effects including a mild lowering of the blood pressure, septic infection from the injection, incorrect insertion of the needle causing respiratory paralysis, or loss of control of the bladder, requiring cathetarization.

Acupuncture, on the other hand, is only mildly invasive and can be quite effective for relieving pain during labor. There are points on various parts of the body where needles can be placed and a woman may not even notice their presence. I have even heard of a case where acupuncture was so successful that the woman had almost no discomfort at all until the needles were removed during the final stage of delivery!

Initiating or Speeding Labor

Acupuncture is commonly used to initiate labor that is significantly late or has started and then stopped, or to hasten it in cases where it has slowed to the point that nothing is really happening. This is useful because many Western obstetricians will decide upon a Caesarean delivery in cases where the child is more than 2 weeks overdue or if the amniotic sac has broken but labor has yet to begin or is not progressing.

In cases where labor has begun and then slowed or stopped, the woman may become so exhausted that the labor becomes progressively more difficult for her. The more fatigued a woman is, the more painful the labor is apt to become and the more likely there is to be the use of pain medications, spinal nerve blockers, or other, progressively more aggressive intervention. When possible, it is better to use the minor interventions of acupuncture and/or herbal therapy during labor than to end up with a complex and potentially dangerous delivery or a C-section.

Herbal tonics may be used to keep up a woman's strength and vitality during labor, and acupuncture or acupressure massage may be used to lessen the discomfort of contractions. Both are quite effective during labor.

Retention of the Placenta

Another possible complication during labor is retention of the placenta. Chinese medicine says that this may happen for one of two reasons: either the qi has been depleted by pregnancy and labor to the point that it cannot expel anything else after the child comes out, or there is blood stasis in the pelvis which keeps the placenta from moving. In old China, this blood stasis was believed to be caused by an invasion of cold into the uterus. In our times, this is less apt to be case. Most blood stasis causing retention of the placenta is a further development of qi stagnation, stagnant dampness, or traumatic injury that does not allow the blood to flow properly. Acupuncture may be quite effective in relieving this condition. It is usually the treatment of first choice since it is simple and immediate. If acupuncture is not immediately effective, there are herbal prescriptions that can be used. These require the cooking of bulk herbs and are, therefore, more time consuming, but are usually effective.

Hemorrhaging During Labor

Hemorrhaging during labor is also not uncommon and is seen by both Western and Chinese medicine to be potentially serious. In Chinese medicine, hemorrhaging during or at the end of labor is usually due to qi emptiness or vacuity. Either the qi has been so depleted by the strain of labor or was already so weak before labor began that it can no longer perform its function of restraining the blood within its vessels. This can be treated effectively, usually by herbal medicine, but it must be treated quickly or Western medical intervention must usually be sought.

It is important to emphasize again that problems which may arise during labor are, like problems during pregnancy or any other time, different in each woman, even if they have the same Western named diagnosis. Three cases of retained placenta (or morning sickness, or postpartum fatigue) may have three different Chinese medical diagnoses requiring three different sets of acupuncture points or three different herbal formulas. Each woman must be assessed individually, since a named Western disease or condition may have several different pattern diagnoses in Chinese medicine.

Postpartum Recuperation

I mmediately after labor, a new mother will typically be exhilarated and exhausted simultaneously. Although not always the case, the most common Chinese medical imbalance occurring immediately after labor and delivery is exhaustion or vacuity of qi and/or blood. This can manifest in a number of ways. The level of postpartum qi or blood exhaustion is dependent upon the prenatal health of the mother, the difficulty and length of her labor, and the amount and duration of blood loss during labor.

If possible, immediately after the labor, the mother should rest or sleep if she can. During this time the father or another family member may hold, rock, sing to, and otherwise bond with the newborn child. This may be difficult in some hospital situations but. However, due to consumer pressure, most Western hospitals are much less stiff and regulated in their birthing and neonatal practices than they were 20 years ago. In any case, the mother should rest as best she can.

During the first few weeks or the first month, she should rest and sleep whenever possible and not be required to return to her work or household duties unless no other options are available. Either family members should take over the new mother's household duties or help should be brought in. In some areas, there are now services specializing in cooking and cleaning for newly delivered mothers.

Other than the immediate care and feeding of the newborn, her schedule should not be too regulated or restricted. Walks in the fresh air are appropriate, but no vigorous exercise or overwork is thought to be wise at this time according to traditional Chinese medicine.

73

Such rest and freedom from responsibility can go a long way toward speeding a woman's recuperation without any other specific intervention.

Postpartum Diet

In China it is an old folk custom for new mothers to be fed with rich, greasy, high nutrient, and high protein foods in the first weeks following delivery. While such foods are recuperative and nutritious, too much of them can cause the production of dampness and phlegm in the body. This can lead to other problems that we have already discussed above.

The basic thing to remember is that pregnancy and labor use very large amounts of qi and blood. Further, breast milk is made from blood as well. For a woman's qi and blood to return to normal after pregnancy and labor, and for her to maintain healthy milk production, her spleen and stomach need continual support during the year or so after her child is born. This is true even if she stops breast feeding sooner than that. Thus, most women should stay on the same type of diet that was suggested in the chapter on self-care. This includes mostly cooked, fresh vegetables, grains, noodles, soups and stews, breads, some animal protein, and a small amount of fruit. We should remember that this type of diet is the one on which humans have evolved over the last several millennia. It is a basic, moderate approach to diet for anyone living in a temperate climate.[1] Beyond that, specific suggestions about diet should be made in consultation

---

[1]   For anyone interested in a more specific description of healthy diet according to Chinese medicine, I suggest reading *Arisal of the Clear: A Simple Guide to Healthy Eating According to Traditional Chinese Medicine*, by Bob Flaws, Blue Poppy Press, ISBN 0-936185-27-9, $8.95

with one's Chinese medical practitioner based upon a woman's constitution and condition.

Postpartum Discharge or Lochia

The lochia is the blood that continues to flow from a woman for several days or even a few weeks after a child is born. In Chinese medicine, this discharge is considered very important since, during birth, a woman's entire body is at its most open and able to discharge. While the qi and blood of a newly birthed mother may require supplementation and support, it is not wise to cut off the valuable opportunity for discharge that the lochia provides. This is a delicate balance between discharge and supplementation and requires some attention and care from the practitioner.

If the lochia is dark and clotty and if there is pain in the lower abdomen, it is very important for blood stasis to be discharged from the uterus with Chinese herbs. However, if the lochia is pale and watery and goes on too long or is too voluminous, one should supplement the qi. These distinctions are important. If one wrongly supplements when they should have eliminated stasis postpartum, this may aggravate the woman's immediate condition and cause long-term complications. Therefore, the postpartum management of the lochia deserves care and attention by a well-trained and experienced practitioner.

Postpartum Problems

It may often be that a woman has an easy pregnancy and labor only to experience health problems after her child in born. While the Chinese medical pattern description of these problems may be different from the named diseases and conditions of Western medicine, Chinese medicine is, nonetheless, quite effective at dealing with most women's postpartum issues. Some postpartum difficulties for which a woman might seek a practitioner of Chinese medicine include postpartum insomnia, fainting or dizziness, abdominal pain, depression, fatigue, constipation, incontinence, fever, or problems with the flow of milk, to name only the most common. There are effective treatments for all th ese problems in the Chinese medical repertoire. Several of them deserve specific discussion.

Postpartum insomnia

Sleep depends on adequate yin (substance: blood, liquids, *jing*) in the body. Consciousness or wakefulness are yang (function: qi, warmth, movement, spirit) Yang must be enfolded or rooted in yin for sleep to occur. If yin becomes insufficient in the body, yang may lose its root and come out of balance, keeping the body awake when it should be asleep. The most common cause of this is blood and fluid loss during labor and/or blood vacuity due to breastfeeding (since milk is made from blood and liquids). Therefore, the main treatments for postpartum insomnia focus on nourishing and supplementing yin and blood, allowing yang to be rebalanced and the spirit to come to rest.

There are other possible factors that may also cause or participate in causing this problem, but the disease mechanisms are complex to explain in a book of this kind. Therefore, women with postpartum insomnia should seek qualified care from a practitioner of Chinese medicine.

Postpartum depression

A survey of 72,000 American women published in the November 1992 issue of *Parents Magazine* said that 53.8% of women experience some degree of postpartum depression. However, what we call postpartum depression can mean many different things in different women. This may include anxiety and restlessness, fright and heart palpitations, anger and frustration, confusion and loss of memory, or extreme fatigue with feelings of hopelessness.

While Chinese medicine has no exact disease counterpart, these types of problems are discussed in Chinese medicine under the category of postpartum palpitations, vexation, and abstraction. Among the symptoms are: clouding of the memory, lack of heart spirit tranquility, confused or chaotic speech, vexation, agitation, restless fidgeting, and insomnia. This is believed to be caused by excessive blood loss during delivery, leaving the heart empty of qi and blood. When the heart is empty of qi and blood there is no place for the heart spirit to rest. The situation is similar to what is described above under postpartum insomnia.

What one may notice here is that there is no separation between mental/emotional symptoms and physical symptoms in Chinese medicine. A healthy mental/emotional state is nothing other than a reflection of healthy body, healthy relationships between the organs, and sufficient and smoothly flowing qi, blood, *jing*, and liquids. Various aspects of one's mental/emotional make-up are closely related to each organ. The health of the psyche is, therefore, a direct reflection of the proper functioning of the organs. Thus, there are no specific *psychological* treatments for postpartum depression in Chinese medicine. There are, however, acupuncture and herbal therapies which, by addressing organ and/or substance imbalances, effectively treat psychoemotional imbalances simult aneously.

It is important to note here that there may also be sociological or economic factors involved in what we call postpartum depression. For one thing, modern Western culture and community structures can be quite isolating for a new mother. She may not have the support of a village, a tribe, or even of her immediate family, thus making her feel quite alone. Secondly, if she is unable to take the first month after her baby's birth for rest and freedom from scheduled responsibilities, she may not recuperate her qi and blood to a healthy level. If her body is still depleted when she returns to her job, or whatever other duties she may have, she may easily feel fatigued and overwhelmed. This leaves her prone to some of the symptoms described above.

Finally, it is important to remember the role that liver stagnation may play in the scenario of postpartum depression. You may remember that, in the first chapter on Chinese medical terminology and theory, I explained that the liver is responsible for the smooth and regular flow of qi throughout the body. If the smooth and even flow of qi is interrupted because the liver is constrained or its qi is stagnated, one may experience this emotionally as frustration, feelings of stuckness, anger, or depression. The liver is called "the temperamental organ" in Chinese medicine, which means that it is the organ most affected by stress. What this means, unfortunately, is that the most common reasons for the liver to become constrained or stagnant in the first place are those same feelings of frustration, anger, or any negative emotional stress for which a woman has no solution, no outlet, nor the ability to change. Thus, there is the possibility of a self-perpetuating cycle which, once begun, can be difficult to break. Add to this fatigue, lack of sleep, and overwork, and it is easy to see how postpartum depression may arise.

While acupuncture and Chinese herbal medicine can be very effective in helping a woman break this cycle, a woman must also help herself with proper self-care. That means regular relaxation and rest, proper diet to help restore the qi and blood, adequate sleep to calm the spirit, mild, regular exercise to circulate the qi, and emotional support from family and friends.

Breastfeeding

The advantages and importance of breastfeeding have been discussed in great detail in many books on pregnancy and mothering, and more American women are breastfeeding their children. According to a recent study reported in the November 1992 issue of *Parents Magazine*, 75% of American women breastfeed their babies for at least some time. Both the mother and child benefit physically and psychologically from breastfeeding. Breast milk is the perfect food for the child. It is provided by nature at the correct temperature, with the appropriate mix of nutrients for a human infant's needs, and antibodies to protect the child from infection.

For the woman, breastfeeding is important since the body is geared up and ready to produce the milk. By aborting the production chemically, it is possible to produce stagnation of qi, blood, and dampness in the breast tissues, which can cause problems later. Many studies over the last 20 years indicate that there is a very direct correlation between breastfeeding and lower incidences of cancer. Chinese medical theory supports this information because breastfeeding encourages the open and free flow of the qi and blood in the breast, thus preventing stagnation. Further, the suckling of the child in the first days after delivery will help the uterus and vagina to contract and return to their normal size.

For both mother and child, breastfeeding offers a time for bonding, quiet time that our modern life does not often allow. It also gives time to continue the close physical tie that will remain between them for many months or even years. From a preventive point of view, the most important things for a woman to keep in mind *vis à vis* breast-feeding are proper nutrition and proper hygiene.

It takes blood to make milk and qi to make blood. Therefore the same dietary suggestions that we made for pregnant women remain important for lactating women, since the basis of qi and blood production rest with the spleen and stomach. Also, breastfeeding requires many more calories than a woman would otherwise need. Therefore, she must be sure to get adequate nutrition so that her own body does not become depleted. The first few months of breastfeeding is not the best time to go on a diet.

Women should keep their breasts and nipples clean between feedings to eliminate the possibility of infection and to prevent the possibility of milk drying and clogging the milk ducts in the nipples.

Problems sometime do arise with breastfeeding, even when a woman is doing everything right. The most common problems are discussed below. All may be treated with Chinese medicine if self-care measures are ineffective.

Agalactia

Agalactia or failure to produce enough milk has two basic causes. First, there may not be enough qi and blood available to produce the milk. This, in turn, may be due to insufficiency of spleen qi and/or severe blood loss during delivery. If this is the case, there may also be dizziness, lack of appetite, insomnia, ringing in the ears, and other symptoms of qi and blood vacuity. The best way for a woman to help herself if she has this condition is to eat as nourishing a diet as possible to try and generate more qi and blood.

In the second type of agalactia, the milk is there but it cannot flow.

This, in turn, is due to stagnation of qi and blood causing a stoppage of the milk. Usually this is at least partially due to liver qi stagnation as described above, since the liver channel flows to the nipples and through the chest area. It is important for such women to relax as completely as possible while breastfeeding and to try to find effective methods of dealing with their stress or other negative emotions.

Galactorrhea

This word describes an incessant flow of milk, which does not stop when the child stops sucking. If a postpartum woman has a strong constitution and her qi and blood are flourishing, even if her breasts are distended and the breast milk is overflowing, this is considered normal and should not be treated with herbal prescriptions. If she is frail, thin, weak, fatigued, or pale, there may be insufficient qi which cannot hold the milk within its vessels. Other symptoms may include a pale complexion, fatigue, cold limbs, watery stools, or frequent urination.

The other possible cause is that the liver is stagnant and overheated. Here one might think of a pan on the stove in which one is heating milk. If the heat is too high, the milk will boil over the top of the pan and overflow. This is very much what happens when the liver becomes overheated. In this case, the woman may also be constipated, nervous and agitated, with scant, dark yellow urine, and swelling or pain in the breasts.

Mastitis

Mastitis is an inflammation of the breasts during lactation. There may be a lumpy or hard area within the breast, accompanied by pain, swelling, heat, and redness. There may or may not be a fever. This is usually due, at least partially, to the excessive ingestion of rich,

81

fatty foods causing the stomach to become overheated. There may also be emotional disturbance and agitation causing the liver to become stagnant and overheated. While the stomach channel irrigates the breast tissue, the liver channel flows directly to the nipples. Both liver and stomach may be involved.

Before having mastitis, a woman may have had agalactia that was due to liver qi stagnation causing the milk to stop flowing. If this stagnation lasts for a while, the qi, which is inherently warm in nature, will overheat the breast tissue. The heat dries the fluids out of the milk. What is left over becomes hard and lumpy, unable to flow through the milk ducts.

It is also possible that mastitis may be caused by an external invasion of wind cold or wind heat which invades the channels in the breasts, blocking the normal flow of milk. Acupuncture and herbal medicine can usually take care of this quite quickly. Such invasions by external pathogens are typically the result of postpartum insufficiency in turn due to loss of qi and blood during labor.

While Chinese herbs and acupuncture can be helpful in all these cases, it is important for a woman to improve her diet, cutting down on rich foods that may be culprits. If emotional problems are causing her liver to become stagnant, she also needs to address these if she can. Remedially, she may use hot compresses before and during breastfeeding. Continuing to breast feed through the affected breast is encouraged as it helps open the blockage causing the pain. This will not cause harm to the child.

Cracked Nipples

Some breastfeeding women experience cracking, chapping, pain, and itching of their nipples. In the Chinese medical literature, this condition is usually not discussed in gynecology texts but is categorized as a dermatological condition. It is quite common for the baby of a woman with this condition to have thrush. In premodern texts, the condition is called nipple wind. It is most commonly seen in primaparas, or first time mothers.

Women with this condition, which is fungal in microbial origin, should decrease their sugar and sweet intake, including fruits and fruit juices and eat less refined carbohydrates. In particular, they should avoid yeasted and fermented products such as risen breads, vinegar, and alcohol.

Getting Back in Shape

During a normal, vaginal delivery, the vagina stretches to accommodate the child's emerging body. After delivery, the suckling of the child begins the process of returning the uterus and vagina to normal size. However, there are things that a woman can do to help this process. During the first few weeks after delivery, exercise should not be excessive or strenuous. A woman can go a long way toward getting her body back in shape by beginning a minimal program of exercise designed to tighten the vagina, return the stomach to its normal muscle tone, and return the uterus to its proper shape and position.

Some midwives suggest that tiny "situps" should begin as soon as one or two days after delivery. These involve just lifting the head off the floor with the knees bent comfortably up. Kegel exercises are also advisable, almost from the very first day after delivery. A Kegel exercise is a contraction of the vaginal and perineal muscles[2]. Some books suggest that the contraction should not include the anus, but I personally find this very difficult to do. In any case, the contraction should be held for 20-30 seconds and then released, with 40 to 100 repetitions of the exercise at least once per day for several weeks or months after delivery.

There are several books available which describe these and other useful, simple exercises for both pregnant women and new mothers. I highly recommend that women find a book like this to help them get back into shape after pregnancy. This is not for cosmetic purposes alone, but also for the long term health of the organs and other body tissues. See the Suggested Reading section in the back of this book for details.

Chinese medicine also has several herbal formulas for vaginal washes or suppositories to tighten and strengthen the vagina. Internal herbs can be used if a woman has feelings of falling or pressing down of her uterus or vagina. She should ask her practitioner about these if problems getting back in shape arise.

In terms of weight loss after the birth of a child, extra weight a woman has gained often disappears with breastfeeding. Breastfeeding requires many more calories than most women's normal diet. Although excessive eating will cause problems, a newly birthed, breastfeeding mother should not immediately go on a diet even if she feels she is carrying more weight than she wants. The best thing for

---

[2]   This pelvic floor exercise was developed by Dr. Arnold Kegel, and is one of the most important exercises for women during and after pregnancy. For further detail, see *A Complete Beauty, Health, & Energy Guide to the Nine Months of Pregnancy, and the Nine Months After* by Wende Devlin Gates and Gail McFarland Meckel, 1980, Viking Press, p. 118-119

a woman to do is to eat a proper diet that supports the spleen and stomach and the creation of qi and blood. If there is plenty of qi, then liquids will be properly transformed and dampness will not accumulate in the body as fat. Any excessive weight gain during pregnancy may very well take care of itself quite naturally.

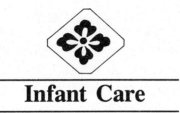

Infant Care

T here are many fine books available on infant and neonatal care, and this book is mostly about caring for your infant during pregnancy rather than after delivery. There are, however, a few key ideas that Chinese medicine can add concerning the care and feeding of infants. The most important of these concerns diet. Of the many ways in which an infant or small child differs from an adult, the most significant is that their digestion is inherently weak. Because of this inherent weakness or immaturity of digestion, Chinese medicine believes that almost all pediatric diseases of children under the age of six begin with some element of indigestion.

To illustrate this, let us take the example of an internal combustion engine. If not functioning at full capacity, an engine will by unable to properly burn all the gasoline that is put in it. Incomplete combustion of gasoline leads to engine sludge.

Something like this process happens in humans, and even more often in human babies. The process of digestion is like combustion. Food and liquids are transformed into qi and blood by a process of warm transformation. When one's digestive fire is weak or inadequate to the task, it is very common for the digestion of the food to be incomplete. There is simply not enough heat to completely "burn up" or transform all the food. The incomplete combustion of food in the body also leads to sludge, or dampness and phlegm.

Chinese medicine says that the child's tiny digestive organs are not fully mature and are inherently weak. This makes them even mo re prone to the creation of phlegm. In Chinese medicine, it is said that "the spleen is the root of phlegm production, but the lungs are the storehouse of phlegm." What this means in practical terms is that incomplete digestion and an inherently weak spleen lead to the creation of turbid dampness in the body that congeals into phlegm and then lodges in the lungs. Mothers see this in their babies as runny noses, productive, phlegmy coughs, ear infections, and other respiratory difficulties.

What this means in terms of prevention is a well-regulated diet, and not over-feeding one's child. This usually means some form of feeding schedule and not feeding on demand. The reason for this is to allow the baby's immature and inefficient digestion time to do its job. Over-feeding a baby is like pouring food that it cannot digest on top of food that has not yet been digested. This also assumes that the baby is growing normally and the breast milk is of sufficient quantity.

I realize that this dictum of scheduled feeding is controversial. It goes against the advice of some women's and mothers' organizations who support feeding on demand for emotional nurturance and other reasons. While I do support holding, rocking, singing, carrying, and massaging one's infant on demand as much as possible, the experience of Chinese medicine suggests that feeding on demand is not the best idea. For mothers interested in a more detailed account of pediatric dietary theory, I refer the reader to *Food, Phlegm, and Pediatric Disease* by Bob Flaws, a small pamphlet for parents, which is listed in the Suggested Reading section in the back.

The other important suggestion for prevention of disease in infants is regular, even daily preventive massage, done by the parents, preferably the father. I suggest this because it gives the father a chance to bond with the child physically in the early days and weeks in a way that he may not otherwise have. The mother is more likely to be the person who is responsible for the feeding, bathing, changing, and minute to minute physical care of the child. Spending the 15-

30 minutes that an infant massage requires gives the father a chance to participate quite directly and meaningfully in his baby's care, and the benefits are enormous. The child will have increased circulation of qi and blood, improved resistance to disease, better sleeping and eating habits, better socialization, better coordination, and an improved disposition. There are several good books available on infant massage and it is not difficult to learn.[3] Babies love massage, even strong and vigorous strokes and, until they reach the busy crawling stages, look forward to this part of their day. If an ounce of prevention is worth a pound of cure, infant massage is the perfect example.

---

[3]   Blue Poppy Press has published a new book in Chinese infant massage, *Chinese Pediatric Massage Therapy*, for both remedial and preventive care. It is an excellent resource for new parents wishing to play a direct role in the health and well-being of their baby.

Finding a Practitioner
of Chinese Medicine

Traditional Chinese medicine is a rapidly rising star within the American alternative health care community. As of this writing, there are more than 25 American schools and colleges of acupuncture and Chinese medicine. That means that the number of professional American practitioners of this art is growing by about five hundred practitioners per year. Many American practitioners have also either gone to medical school in Asia or have gone to Asia for post-graduate training. And, of course, many Asian doctors have immigrated to the United States in the last twenty years.

In addition, there is a National Council of Acupuncture Schools and Colleges, which helps to oversee and regulate the quality of training and education. The National Commission for the Certification of Acupuncturists helps to insure minimum, entry level, professional competence. The various state and national professional associations, such as the National Acupuncture and Oriental Medicine Alliance, help to regulate professional ethics, network among practitioners, and provide continuing, post-graduate education. Acupuncture has now been legalized as a state-approved healthcare modality in over a score of states and, in many others, favorable legislation is in the process of being enacted.

In states where acupuncture is licensed and state-regulated, one should be able to find the names of local practitioners in the yellow pages of the phone book or by contacting the state Department of Health, Board of Medical Examiners, or Department of Regulatory Agencies. In such states, it is wise to insure that potential practitioners are state licensed. In states without licensure, it is best to seek out those practitioners who are nationally board certified. Such practitioners typically append the initials Dipl. Ac., for Diplomate of Acupuncture, after their names. These national board exams insure minimal professional competency and not less than the equivalent of two full years of academic and clinical training specifically in acupuncture.

In the United States, not all acupuncturists are practitioners of Chinese herbal medicine, but almost without exception, all American practitioners of Chinese herbal medicine are also acupuncturists. As yet, only a handful of states include Chinese herbal education and examination in their licensing. Recently, the National Commission for the Certification of Acupuncturists has begun the process of creating an exam for national herbal certification. Therefore, it is important to query potential practitioners on the school, nature, and extent of their Chinese herbal training. In general, the practice of Chinese internal or herbal medicine is more demanding and requires more education and experience than the practice of acupuncture.

When searching out a qualified and knowledgeable practitioner, satisfied, word-of-mouth referrals are important. It is also appropriate to ask for references to previous patients treated for the same problem. Likewise, it is important that the practitioner be able to communicate with the patient in order to explain their Chinese diagnosis and the rationale behind their treatment plan. In all cases, a professional practitioner of Chinese medicine should be able and willing to give a written traditional Chinese diagnosis of the patient's case. Also, I personally suggest that patients select practitioners who belong to both local and national Chinese medicine/acupuncture professional associations. Such associations offer referrals of professional members in good standing and high repute. In addition, such associations usually have a code of professional ethics that their members promise to uphold. This further insures the quality and professionalism of the care they provide.

Traditional Chinese medicine, including acupuncture, is a discrete and independent health care profession. It is not a technique to be added to the bag of tricks of some other profession. It takes just as long *or longer* to learn Chinese medicine as it does to learn allopathy, chiropractic, naturopathy, or homeopathy. Previous training in one of these systems in no way confers *a priori* competence or knowledge in Chinese medicine or acupuncture. Therefore, I heartily advise prospective patients seeking to avail themselves of the benefits of traditional Chinese medicine to seek out professionally trained practitioners of this system. As suggested above, just as one would not hire a plumber to do electrical wiring, so patients should receive Chinese medicine from professionally trained practitioners of Chinese medicine.

For further information regarding the American practice of Chinese medicine and acupuncture and for referrals to local professional associations and practitioners, prospective patients may contact:

> National Commission for the Certification of
> Acupuncturists
> 1424 16th St. N.W., Suite 501
> Washington, D.C. 20036
> (202) 232-1404

or:

> National Acupuncture and Oriental Medicine Alliance
> 638 Prospect Ave.
> Hartford, CT 06105-4298
> (203) 586-7550

Conclusion

I deally, pregnancy is a time when a woman should feel at the peak of her strength and health, emotionally centered and well. While almost every pregnant woman has some discomforts and some fears or worries, her basic good health should help her to overcome these with relative ease. This book is written to help pregnant women achieve these goals and to inform them that Chinese medicine offers an alternative route to arriving at and maintaining this state of health and wellbeing.

While many Americans may have heard of acupuncture through various news media, Chinese medicine as a whole system of medicine remains largely unknown and untried by the majority. Few are aware of the scope of its understanding of human suffering, the breadth of its treatment options, or its level of effectiveness as an alternative or complement to Western medical therapies.

Because of its effectiveness in the field of gynecology, Chinese medicine is an option of which Western women should be made aware. Also, because the emphasis is on prevention and the maintenance of long term health, Chinese medicine has much to offer women before, during, and after pregnancy and throughout life.[1]

It is my primary purpose in writing this book to inform women about what Chinese medicine can do for them and their babies during the childbearing year. At a time in American history when there has been so much political focus on the family, it is my desire to bring some

---

[1]   For information about other books on women's health care and Chinese medicine by this author, see the Suggested Reading section.

of Chinese medicine's wisdom and compassion about this most important family event to women in the West. It is my hope that this small volume may inspire women to seek Chinese medical care at this time in their lives or any ti me they need health care advice. For those of you reading this book who are pregnant or who are planning to become pregnant soon, I heartily wish you a healthy pregnancy and healthy baby.

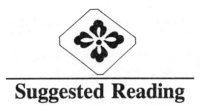

Suggested Reading

Books on Chinese Medicine

The Web That Has No Weaver Ted Kaptchuk, Congdon & Weed, 1983. General introduction to Chinese medical theories.

Arisal of the Clear: A Simple Guide to Healthy Eating According to Chinese Medicine Bob Flaws, Blue Poppy Press, 1991.

Menopause, A Second Spring: Making a Smooth Transition with Traditional Chinese Medicine Honora Lee Wolfe, Blue Poppy Press, 1992

Food, Phlegm, and Pediatric Disease: A Guide to the Care & Feeding of Infants According To Chinese Medicine a pamphlet by Bob Flaws, Blue Poppy Press, 1989

Chinese Pediatric Massage Therapy: A Parent's & Practitioner's Guide to the Treatment and Prevention of Childhood Disease by Fan Ya-li, Blue Poppy Press, 1994

The Treatment of Children by Acupuncture, Julian Scott, Journal of Chinese Medicine, Hove, Sussex, UK, 1986

General Books on Natural Health for Women

Alternative Health Care Resources: A Directory & Guide Brett Jason Sinclair, Parker Publishing Co., 1992

Mayo Clinic Family Health Book, Morrow Publishing, 1991

The Complete Guide to Women's Health Bruce D. Shepard, MD, and

The Complete Guide to Women's Health Bruce D. Shepard, MD, and Carroll A. Shephard, RN, PhD.

Natural Healing for Women: Caring for Yourself With Herbs, Homeopathy, & Essential Oils Susan Curtis & Romy Frazier, Pandora Press, 1991

The Art of Good Living - Simple Steps to Regaining Health & the Joy of Life Svevo Brooks, Houghton Mifflin, 1990

Books on Pregnancy, Babies, and Birthing

The American Way of Birth Jessica Mitford, Dutton, Penguin Group, 1992

Special Delivery Rahima Baldwin, Celestial Arts, 1986

Active Birth - The New Approach to Giving Birth Naturally Janet Balaskas, Hartford Common Press, 1992

Babies Remember Birth & Other Extraordinary Scientific Discoveries About The Mind & Personality of Your Newborn by David Chamberlain PhD, Ballantine, 1988

Communing With the Spirit of Your Unborn Child Dawson Church, Aslan Publishing, 1988

Silent Knife: Cesarean Prevention & Vaginal Birth After Cesarean Nancy Warner Cohen & Lois J. Estner, Bergen & Garvey Publishers, 1983

The Secret Life of the Unborn Child: How You Can Prepare Your Unborn Baby for a Happy, Healthy Life Thomas Verny, MD, with John Kelly, A Delta Book, Dell Publishing, 1981

Mother Massage — A Handbook for Relieving the Discomforts of Pregnancy Elaine Stillerman, LMT, Delta Books, Dell Publishing, 1992

Books on Pre and Postnatal Exercise

Elisabeth Bing's Guide to Moving Through Pregnancy Noonday Press, 1991

Positive Pregnancy Fitness: A Guide to a More Comfortable Pregnancy & Easier Birth Through Exercise & Relaxation Sylvia Klein Olkin, MS, Avery Publishing Group, 1987

The Postnatal Exercise Book - A Program of Fitness & Well Being for Mother & Baby Margie Polden & Barbara Whiteford, Barron's Education Series, Inc., 1992

Jane Fonda's New Pregnancy & Total Birth Program: A Comprehensive Guide to the Physical & Emotional Aspects of Pregnancy, Birth, & Recovery, by Emmy DeLyser, A Fireside Book from Simon & Schuster, 1989

Index

A

abdominal pain 25, 55, 56, 76
abdominal pain, severe 25
acid regurgitation 63
activity, vigorous 25
acupuncture 5, 26-28, 48-50, 54-56, 62, 70-73, 78, 79, 82, 95, 91-93, 97
agalactia 80-82
agitation 58, 64, 77, 82
albuminuria 61, 62
ankles, edema in the 48
antibiotic-free 39
aphonia 62

B

baby, malformed 59
bao gong 8, 11
bao mai 10, 11, 34
birth defects 16
birth, hasten or smooth the process of 65
blood and yin, production of 15
blood loss, excessive 77
blood pressure, high 62, 63
blood stasis 41, 58, 71, 75
bowels, dampness and heat in the 61
bowels, hollow 8, 9
breast milk is overflowing 81
breastfeeding 76, 79-84
breasts, inflammation of the 81

C

Caesarean section 63, 66-69
calcium 38, 39
cathetarization 70

charity 34
chicken pox 31
Chinese herbal medicine 49-51, 56, 59-62, 79, 92
chong mai 10, 12, 34, 58
chorioadenoma 55
cinnabar field 29
cold injury 61, 63
common cold 63
conception 7, 8, 10, 13, 19-21, 23, 31
constipation 33, 42, 76
contemplation 34
contraction 27, 84
convulsions 63
cough 55, 61
coughs, phlegmy 88
cravings 39, 40

D

dampness 13, 38-40, 42, 54, 60-62, 72, 74, 79, 85, 87, 88
diarrhea 55, 61
dietary regulation 26, 42
digestion, immaturity of 87
digestion, inefficient 88
digestion, impaired 61
digestive organs, tiny 87
discharge of toxins 37
discrimination of diseases 53
disease, chronic 57, 60
disease, improved resistance to 89
disposition, improved 89
dizziness 55, 76, 80
Down's syndrome 16
dry-brushing 44
dysentery 55
dysphoria 55

101

SOMETHING OLD, SOMETHING NEW; Essays on the TCM Description of Western Herbs, Pharmaceuticals, Vitamins & Minerals by Bob Flaws ISBN 0-936185-21-X $19.95

A NEW AMERICAN ACUPUNCTURE: Acupuncture Osteopathy, by Mark Seem, ISBN 0-936185-44-9, $19.95

SCATOLOGY & THE GATE OF LIFE: The Role of the Large Intestine in Immunity, An Integrated Chinese-Western Approach by Bob Flaws ISBN 0-936185-20-1 $14.95

MENOPAUSE, A Second Spring: Making A Smooth Transition with Traditional Chinese Medicine by Honora Lee Wolfe ISBN 0-936185-18-X $14.95

MIGRAINES & TRADITIONAL CHINESE MEDICINE: A Layperson's Guide by Bob Flaws ISBN 0-936185-15-5 $11.95

STICKING TO THE POINT: A Rational Methodology for the Step by Step Administration of an Acupuncture Treatment by Bob Flaws ISBN 0-936185-17-1 $16.95

ENDOMETRIOSIS & INFERTILITY AND TRADITIONAL CHINESE MEDICINE: A Laywoman's Guide by Bob Flaws ISBN 0-936185-14-7 $9.95

THE BREAST CONNECTION: A Laywoman's Guide to the Treatment of Breast Disease by Chinese Medicine by Honora Lee Wolfe ISBN 0-936185-13-9 $9.95

NINE OUNCES: A Nine Part Program For The Prevention of AIDS in HIV Positive Persons by Bob Flaws ISBN 0-936185-12-0 $9.95

THE TREATMENT OF CANCER BY INTEGRATED CHINESE-WESTERN MEDICINE by Zhang Dai-zhao, trans. by Zhang Ting-liang ISBN 0-936185-11-2 $18.95

A HANDBOOK OF TRADITIONAL CHINESE DERMATOLOGY by Liang Jian-hui, trans. by Zhang Ting-liang & Bob Flaws, ISBN 0-936185-07-4 $15.95

A HANDBOOK OF TRADITIONAL CHINESE GYNECOLOGY by Zhejiang College of TCM, trans. by Zhang Ting-liang, ISBN 0-936185-06-6 (2nd edit.) $21.95

PRINCE WEN HUI'S
COOK: Chinese Dietary
Therapy by Bob Flaws &
Honora Lee Wolfe, ISBN 0-
912111-05-4, $12.95 (Published by
Paradigm Press, Brookline, MA)

THE DAO OF
INCREASING LONGEVITY
AND CONSERVING ONE'S
LIFE by Anna Lin & Bob Flaws,
ISBN 0-936185-24-4 $16.95

FIRE IN THE VALLEY:
The TCM Diagnosis and
Treatment of Vaginal
Diseases by Bob Flaws
ISBN 0-936185-25-2 $16.95

HIGHLIGHTS OF
ANCIENT ACUPUNCTURE
PRESCRIPTIONS trans. by
Honora Lee Wolfe & Rose
Crescenz ISBN 0-936185-23-6
$14.95

ARISAL OF THE CLEAR:
A Simple Guide to Healthy
Eating According to
Traditional Chinese Medicine
by Bob Flaws, ISBN #-936185-
27-9 $8.95

PEDIATRIC BRONCHITIS:
ITS CAUSE, DIAGNOSIS &
TREATMENT
ACCORDING TO
TRADITIONAL CHINESE
MEDICINE trans. by Gao Yu-li
and Bob Flaws, ISBN 0-936185-
26-0 $15.95

AIDS & ITS TREATMENT
ACCORDING TO
TRADITIONAL CHINESE
MEDICINE by Huang Bing-
shan, trans. by Fu-Di & Bob
Flaws, ISBN 0-936185-28-7
$24.95

ACUTE ABDOMINAL
SYNDROMES: Their
Diagnosis & Treatment by
Combined Chinese-Western
Medicine by Alon Marcus, ISBN
0-936185-31-7 $16.95

MY SISTER, THE MOON:
The Diagnosis & Treatment
of Menstrual Diseases by
Traditional Chinese Medicine
by Bob Flaws, ISBN 0-936185-
34-1, $24.95

FU QING-ZHU'S
GYNECOLOGY trans. by
Yang Shou-zhong and Liu Da-
wei, ISBN 0-936185-35-X,
$21.95

FLESHING OUT THE
BONES: The Importance of
Case Histories in Chinese
Medicine by Charles Chace.
ISBN 0-936185-30-9, $18.95

CLASSICAL
MOXIBUSTION SKILLS
IN CONTEMPORARY
CLINICAL PRACTICE by
Sung Baek, ISBN 0-936185-16-3
$10.95

MASTER TONG'S ACUPUNCTURE: An Ancient Lineage for Modern Practice, trans. and commentary by Miriam Lee, OMD, ISBN 0-936185-37-6, $19.95

A HANDBOOK OF TCM UROLOGY & MALE SEXUAL DYSFUNCTION by Anna Lin, OMD, ISBN 0-936185-36-8, $16.95

Li Dong-yuan's TREATISE ON THE SPLEEN & STOMACH, A Translation of the *Pi Wei Lun* by Yang Shou-zhong & Li Jian-yong, ISBN 0-936185-41-4, $21.95

PATH OF PREGNANCY, VOL. I, Gestational Disorders by Bob Flaws, ISBN 0-936185-39-2, $16.95

PATH OF PREGNANCY, VOL. II, Postpartum Diseases by Bob Flaws, ISBN 0-936185-42-2, $18.95

How to Have a HEALTHY PREGNANCY, HEALTHY BIRTH with Traditional Chinese Medicine by Honora Lee Wolfe, ISBN 0-936185-40-6, $9.95

MASTER HUA'S CLASSIC OF THE CENTRAL VISCERA by Hua Tuo, translated by Yang Shou-zhong, ISBN 0-936185-43-0, $21.95